Frances Darragh and Louise Darragh Law are cousins. They both lived in Auckland, New Zealand when they first wrote this book. Their experience as natural health practitioners and mothers of young families led to its compilation.

Frances Darragh has degrees in social sciences and anthropology. She is a Registered Natural Health Practitioner specializing in herbs and homoeopathics. She has practised in the natural health field for over ten years. Frances is a member of the New Zealand Association of Counsellors and works as a counsellor in her private practice. With her training and involvement in pre-school education she has a particular interest in children. She also makes time for her passion for music and a growing interest in women's spirituality. She currently lives with her husband and two children in Auckland, New Zealand.

Louise Darragh Law is a qualified Naturopath and Iridologist, and a Registered Homoeopath. She has practised in the natural health field for 15 years, working in clinics in New Zealand and the Australian desert before moving to the UK in 1995. She works in several natural health clinics in Bristol and provides a complete approach to all health problems. One of her specialities is children's health. She is currently studying for a post-graduate diploma in Ayurvedic medicine. In her spare time she writes poetry and is involved in Bristol's performance poetry network. She currently lives with her husband and two of her three children in Bristol, England.

GW00776583

Healing Your Child

An A–Z guide to
safe natural
remedies

Frances Darragh
& Louise Darragh Law

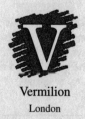

Vermilion
London

1 3 5 7 9 10 8 6 4 2

Text © Frances Darragh & Louise Darragh Law 1989

First published in New Zealand in 1989 by New Women's Press Ltd
A revised and updated edition subsequently published in
New Zealand by Tandem Press, 2 Rugby Road, Birkenhead,
North Shore City, New Zealand

First published in the United Kingdom in 2000 by
Vermilion, an imprint of Ebury Press
Random House, 20 Vauxhall Bridge Road,
London SW1V 2SA

Random House South Africa (Pty) Limited
Endulini, 5A Jubilee Road, Parktown 2193, South Africa

The Random House Group Limited Reg. No. 954009

www.randomhouse.co.uk

A CIP catalogue record for this book is available
from the British Library.

ISBN 0 09 185603 5

Papers used by Vermilion are natural recyclable products
made from wood grown in sustainable forests.

Typeset in Times and Officina Sans
Design/make up by Roger Walker

Printed and bound in Great Britain by
Cox & Wyman Ltd, Reading, Berkshire

PLEASE NOTE

Although every effort has been made to ensure that the contents of this book are accurate, it must not be treated as a substitute for qualified medical advice. Always consult a qualified practitioner. Neither the Author nor the Publishers can be held responsible for any loss or claim arising out of the use, or misuse, of the suggestions made or the failure to take medical advice.

Contents

Foreword

Those of you fortunate enough to use this book are taking a giant step towards self-determination and freedom from the bondage of limited knowledge in child health care. When we become parents we want to do the best job we can. It is not until the baby is in our hands that we become aware just how abysmal our own personal training in child care is, especially in preventing minor health problems from developing into serious ones.

Today's young parents have great pressures placed on them socially to 'do the right thing' for their baby. At the same time, social changes have resulted in grandparents being less available to assist with home remedies and other comforting advice when children are ill. Parents feel isolated and ignorant, yet don't want to run to the doctor with every little thing.

Frances Darragh and Louise Darragh Law are mothers who display a deep sensitivity to the health needs of the community. Their combined talents include Naturopathy, Homoeopathy, Touch for Health and One Brain Instruction. They are living and practising the things that they are writing about. The result is an easy-to-use book full of practical professional advice. Problems requiring medical attention are readily identified so that referring to this book will *not* delay proper advice being sought in an emergency.

Frances and Louise have given parents easy signs and symptoms to help recognize conditions. They then draw on their professional knowledge to provide remedies for those conditions that are easy and *safe* to deal with in the home. Suggestions for seeking the appropriate health professional are also given.

Most of us feel we are just starting to understand child-rearing when our youngest is finishing school. 'I'd like to have known then what I know now' is a common comment. This book does much to remedy that and is the type of book I imagine that women of my mother's generation (born in the 1890s) could well have written, but didn't. We would have referred to it frequently when our girls were growing up.

The essence, then, of this book is its easily understood and practical help. It gives you the answers to a broad spectrum of conditions which form part of the 'mysteries of child health'. I learned things which have added to my capabilities as a parent. You, too, will learn things which, when put to use, will enhance the physical, emotional and mental health of your children. The parenting experience will be less daunting and more rewarding.

BRUCE DEWE

Dr Bruce Dewe is a medical doctor who was for twenty years a family practitioner with a special interest in preventive medicine and health. For many years he has been the South Pacific trainer for the Touch of Health Foundation of the USA, urging people to take more responsibility for their own health care. He and his wife Joan Dewe MA have opened (1988) the Structural Neurology Centre in Auckland, dealing with chronic pain, fears, phobias, obsessions, allergies, dyslexia and other conditions for which conventional medicine has less than adequate answers. Dr and Ms Dewe teach their work throughout the world.

Preface

Dear Reader

We have written this book because we have been in contact with many anxious parents who don't know what to do about their children's health problems. So many times, we have watched parents go off to their medical practitioner only to return with yet another round of antibiotics, no real understanding of what is happening with their child, and a lack of confidence that a solution will be found. We have also watched with grave concern the growing number of children on permanent medication, often requiring an increase in dosage and further medication as new symptoms appear.

We had been through this ourselves as parents and had turned to alternatives. Our partners, children, and pets have put up with some experimentation on behalf of our pursuit but they benefited greatly in the end. In the early days, Andi went off to school with plantain leaves taped to her chin to battle impetigo – experience has taught that there are ways of dealing with such things which require less fortitude from a six-year-old!

After eight ear infections in six months and almost permanent antibiotics, Kelly was of course on the list for the infamous Grommets (tubes in the ears). Though herbs, homoeopathics, Bach Flower Remedies and dietary changes helped, any cold still produced an ear infection. We finally remembered that it had all started with mumps; homoeopathic Nosode finished almost a year's neurosis and motivated us to write a manual for parents like ourselves, in search of alternative remedies.

There are, however, other stories – of Lee whose whooping cough seemed to respond rapidly to the natural approach, while her sister's condition steadily deteriorated despite our using the same methods. Her case of whooping cough demanded hospital care and herbs could only be used to help her convalescence. Nature demands little, and does not always promise miracles.

We respect the need for many aspects of allopathic (orthodox) medicine. However, we also see a great need for caregivers to feel more confident and less useless in both understanding and taking measures to aid the path to health with nature's healers, which are safe if used as directed. The more you use them, the better the body will respond to their action and the more confident you will become.

It is not our intention to replace the services of the physician when such services are obviously required, but rather to complement them. With our alternative approach, parents and caregivers are guided through the progressive stages of illness and the journey back to good health. But if any illness lingers or is in any way serious (we give clear indications for this), it should always be checked and any actions taken monitored carefully by an experienced practitioner. Many medical practitioners are now willing to work *with* caregivers and can give you clear guidelines as to when the often more definitive action of drugs is necessary.

If you are in doubt and feel concerned, the experts are there to be called upon. Be assured – if used as instructed, natural remedies will not inhibit the action of allopathic drugs (although allopathic drugs may render natural remedies useless). Our hope is that the use of natural remedies will not only relieve the world's over-burdened health services and save money for the family in the long run, but, more importantly, will give confidence and control back to the parents, who are so often left coping with and caring for a sick child.

FRANCES DARRAGH & LOUISE DARRAGH LAW

Introduction

This book offers information on how to recognize and act upon children's injuries and ailments, by providing a comprehensive and practical manual. Information is given on the following:

- What symptoms may indicate
- The course an illness usually takes
- What you can do at home
- When to seek professional advice
- How to help the body through its crises in a way that complements any other forms of treatment which the child may be undergoing
- How to prevent a situation from deteriorating to the point where professional advice is essential.

HOW TO USE THIS BOOK

The main text takes the form of an alphabetical guide to children's illnesses. For the convenience of the lay reader and to make the vast symptom picture more accessible, we have compiled information under illness headings rather than specific symptom. Where diagnosis may be difficult, information is listed under the specific parts of the body. A separate section deals with resistance, epidemic diseases and immunization (page 29).

1. For each ailment, we include:
    - The course the illness takes and its possible cause
    - Symptoms to expect
    - What immediate action to follow
    - How to make use of herbs, homoeopathic remedies and cell salts

- When it is vital to call for professional help
- What emergency steps to take before help arrives
- Side-effects, after-effects, or complications
- Follow-up approaches to help convalescence.

2. If you are not sure what illness your child actually has, refer to the index.

3. If you remain at all worried or confused, seek expert advice for diagnosis. Ailments of a doubtful nature or those which are not quickly alleviated belong under expert care, whether natural or orthodox.

USING NATURAL REMEDIES

Detailed instructions on the storage, dosage, usage and combination of natural remedies are given in the following pages. Depending on which kind of remedy you favour, we recommend that you make up a Health Kit to have on hand in your home. Also look to any particular health problems in your family (such as asthma) and have remedies for these in your cabinet. To make your choice of remedy clearer with homoeopathy and cell salts, we provide brief Remedy Pictures at the back of the book as a cross reference.

FIRST AID

We recommend that this book be used in conjunction with a regular First Aid book, such as that published by the St John Ambulance Association. Also see Shock (page 160).

SEEK MEDICAL ADVICE FOR THE FOLLOWING:

Stomach-ache which is getting worse.

Child is distant and confused, with dull eyes.

Child looks anxious or in shock, pale or sweaty.

Sunken eyes, skin lacking elasticity, dry mouth and passing little urine (signs of dehydration).

Neck is stiff and painful to bend or move.

Panting, over-breathing or deep rattling.

Abdominal wall draws in upon breathing.

Breathing difficulty is accompanied by blueness around the mouth.

Blood and mucous appear in stools.

Sharp object embedded in the eye.

Convulsion or fit.

Fracture.

Soreness in kidney region (lower middle of back).

Dark red or smoky urine.

Coughing up blood.

Coma – child can't be wakened.

Sores that don't go away.

Weight loss that continues.

Blood or straw-coloured discharge from the ear.

How to Use Herbs

Herbs can be grown in your garden or be found in most health shops in a variety of forms: fresh, dried, tincture, oil, cough syrup, ointment, bath oil, lotion, capsule, or tablet. All forms are equally acceptable. Your child will quickly let you know which is preferred.

If you wish to produce any of these forms yourself, there are many herbal books describing how to do it.

INTERNAL USE

Herbs contain balanced supplies of nutritional supplements, with an affinity for particular body parts or processes; they work well when taken immediately before or after mealtimes. They can be used singly, but they also work well in combination with each other. Any amount can be combined at once. Hot drinks work best for colds, flu, and chest complaints. They also induce sweating. At other times, herbal drinks may be taken warm or cool. If desired, sweeten drinks with honey when lukewarm (over 45°C/113°F of heat destroys the beneficial properties of honey); if taste is disagreeable, make a syrup (see below).

Dosage: For best results, make up the required amount fresh each day and give 1 tsp to $1/4$ cup three times daily. This can be increased to 2-hourly in acute situations.

The total amount required each day will vary according to the constitution of the child. Use higher amounts for an older child, a stronger constitution, or a more severe disturbance; lower for a younger child, a more sensitive constitution, or more potent herbs (i.e. Hawthorn, Valerian, Lobelia, Jamaica Dogwood, Oats, Stone Root, Senega, Blood Root).

Fresh

For the light-textured parts of the plant (leaves and flowers) and crushed seeds, make as you would a pot of tea: 3 tsp herbs (single or mixed) to 1 cup boiling water. Leave to brew for 10–30 minutes.

Alternatively, mix the same quantities of herbs and cold water, cover, bring to the boil and brew.

For heavy-textured parts of the plant such as bark, stems or roots: 3 tsp herbs (single or mixed) to 1 cup of water, simmer for 15–20 minutes, then strain.

Cold extracts can also be made by leaving the herbs in cold water (in a non-metallic pot) for 8–12 hours.

Dried

It is wise to replenish your supply of dried herbs every twelve months.

For the light-textured parts of the plant (leaves and flowers), make as you would a pot of tea: 1 tsp of herbs (single or mixed) to 1 cup boiling water. Leave to brew 10–30 minutes.

For heavy-textured parts such as bark, stems, and roots: 1 tsp herbs (single or mixed) to 1 cup of water, simmer 15–20 minutes, then strain.

Tincture

The suggested dosage is 6–20 drops (single or mixed) per cup of warm water or juice, depending on the constitution of the child and the severity of the illness. A rule-of-thumb for infant's dosage: one drop per year of age in a small amount of water or milk (up to a quarter of a cup).

Powders

Infants: a pinch to $1/4$ tsp in a half-cup mixed with herb tea or warmed milk. Five to 10 year-olds: $1/4$–$1/2$ tsp in a $1/2$ cup mixed with herb tea or warmed milk.

Herbal Syrup

For coughs, colds and the child who finds the flavour of herb teas disagreeable. Simmer herbs (single or mixed, using the amounts given above) until most of the water has evaporated. Strain and add honey when it is lukewarm.

Capsules and Tablets

These are readily available and directions appear on the packet. If not specified, use half adult dosage for children, quarter adult dosage for under two-year-olds.

EXTERNAL APPLICATIONS

Poultice

The whole fresh leaf can be applied to the area and taped on.
    Alternatively, a poultice may be made as follows:

- Fresh leaves are crushed, bruised or mashed with a little boiling water to soften; or half to 1 tsp of dried leaves are mixed to a paste with bread, milk, wholemeal flour and warm water to soften.

A HERB HEALTH KIT

Barberry *Berberis Vulgaris*
Buchu *Barosoma Betulina*
Burdock *Arctium Lappa*
Cayenne *Capsicum minimum*
Chamomile *Matricaria chamomilla*
Coltsfoot *Tussilago Farfara*
Dandelion Root *Taraxicum officinalis*
Dong Quai *Shi di huang*
Echinacea *Echinacea augustifolia*
Elecampane *Inula helenium*
Eyebright *Euphrasia officinalis*
Gentian *Gentiana lutea*
Golden Seal *Hydrastis canadensis*
Horehound (white) *Marrubium Vulgare*
Irish Moss *Chondrus Crispus*

Juniper *Berries*
Kelp
Liquorice Root *Glycyrrhiza giabra*
Lobelia *Lobelia inflata*
Marigold *Calendula officinalis*
Marshmallow Root *Althea officinalis*
Mullein *Verbascum thapsis*
Myrrh *Commiphorus molmol*
Rhubarb Root *Rheum officinalis*
Rosemary *Rosmarinus officinalis*
Senna Pods *Cassia augustifolia*
Skullcap *Scutellaria lateriflora*
Tansy - *Tanacetum vulgare*
Uva Ursi *Arctostaphylos ura ursi*
Valerian *Valia officinalis*
Yarrow *Achillea milefolium*

There are many herbs other than those we mention which are also of value. For practical purposes, we have limited our list.

- Place the warm herbal mixture between two layers of gauze and apply it to sores, burns, bruises, sprains or strains.
- Cover with a thick padding of towel, blanket or hot-water bottle to retain warmth for as long as possible.

Compress

This is slightly less active than a poultice.

Make a warm cupful of herbs using the amounts given under Internal Use above. Soak a piece of gauze or cloth in this and apply to sores, burns, bruises, sprains or strains. Cover with thick dry towelling, blanket or hot-water bottle to retain warmth for as long as possible. The compress may be moistened with warm water from time to time.

Inhalation

Essential oils make the most effective inhalations, though strong brews may be made of fresh, dried or tincture forms.

Add 1–2 drops of oil to a bowl of steaming water, drape a towel over the head to trap the steam, and breathe deeply into lungs.

Bath

Prepare several herbal cupfuls as directed under Internal Use and add to bath water.

Lotion

Mix herb tincture (5 drops) or herbal oil (2 drops) with $1/2$ cup of Soya or Almond Oil (for dry skin, or as a chest rub); or of Aloe Vera (for irritated skin such as itchy bites or eczema).

Cream

Add 2–3 tsp of herbal tincture to 75 ml jar of acqueous cream. Especially good for surface irritations (calendula or urtica urens) or for bruises (arnica). There are now many ready-made herbal creams available.

How to Use Homoeopathic Remedies

READ THIS CHAPTER

Homoeopathy is a complex and comprehensive system of medicine. The advice we offer here is a simple approach for the lay person. If symptoms continue despite the use of the remedies we suggest, consult an experienced homoeopath who can prescribe from the wide range of remedies through the complex procedure of detailed case-taking.

Homoeopathic remedies are easily obtained from health shops and some chemists (see list, page 215). Some suppliers have a mail order system, so that you can order directly if you have difficulty obtaining remedies locally.

Homoeopathic remedies work on the theory that like cures like, i.e. that a substance which has the ability to cause certain symptoms in a healthy person, can be used to cure those same symptoms in an unhealthy person.

All remedies are alcohol based in tablets: the alcohol is dropped onto lactose tablets.

Tablets are readily available but liquid forms would have to be ordered. It is very unlikely that the amount of alcohol which would be taken in a few doses would have any affect on someone with liver disease.

Remedies can be made from any substance, animal, vegetable or mineral. The process of preparing them involves serial dilution and vigorous shaking to increase the potency of the remedy (and decrease the amount of the material substance). They therefore have few side-effects and are very safe to take in the potency and quantity we recommend.

Store remedies in a cool dark place away from strong odours. Because they are in such minute doses, their effects can be destroyed by excess heat or light, toothpaste, peppermint, strong gargles, camphor, and excess garlic, tea or coffee. Do not touch directly either tablets or droppers.

HOW TO CHOOSE YOUR REMEDY

1. Take note of how your child has changed during the illness, comparing her to how she was when well.
   - How does she look? Anxious? Pale? Glazed eyes? Dry lips?
   - Has her mood changed? Is she irritable? Tearful? Averse to company?
   - Note other characteristics: Does she prefer heat or cold? Is she sweaty? feverish? thirsty? hungry? Does she sit up or lie down? Is she worse at a particular time of the day?

2. Next, using the contents list (and index for guidance if necessary), look up the illness and find the remedy which most closely matches your child's symptoms. If it is difficult to select one particular remedy, look up the Remedy Pictures (page 199). These provide more detailed information about each remedy, and should aid you in your final choice.
   - It is not necessary to have all the symptoms listed under a remedy. Three definite and clear symptoms are often enough.
   - If your chosen remedy causes no reaction after 3 doses, a different remedy may be needed. Retake the case, i.e. check your child's symptoms and check your choice of remedy. Do not change the remedy too often.
   - Traditionally, combining homoeopathic remedies with each other has not been recommended, although it is becoming more common to combine some remedies in low potencies such as 6x or 3c.

3. *Inimicals*. These are remedies which, in some cases, don't follow each other well and cause a negative reaction.
   They are: Apis/Rhus Tox, Phosphorus/Causticum, Silica/ Mercurius, Chamomilla/Nux Vomica, Ignatia/Coffea, Sepia/ Lachesis, Calc Carb/Bryonia, Zinc/Nux Vomica. Follow one with the other *only if absolutely indicated*.

HOW THE REMEDIES ARE TAKEN

Homoeopathic remedies are absorbed into the system via the mucous membranes in the mouth and therefore must be put into a clean mouth with none of the strong flavours mentioned above still lingering. For best results, take no food or drink for half an hour before and after taking the remedy.

Tablets

Children can suck on tablets until dissolved. Administer by tipping tablet into the lid and then directly into the child's mouth or onto a teaspoon and into the mouth so that there is no contact with the fingers.

For babies: crush tablet between two clean metal spoons and either place directly onto baby's tongue or mix with water on teaspoon.

Do not place dropped or touched tablets back into the bottle.

Liquid

Liquid potencies are often in 95% alcohol. This is unpleasant if dropped directly onto the tongue. Place two drops in half a cupful of water, then stir with a metal spoon and the liquid is used as follows: one teaspoon = one dose.

HOW MUCH AND HOW OFTEN

30c Potency

In a sudden crisis: Suck one tablet or take 3–4 drops at each dose. Take a second dose 15 minutes after the first, then double the time between doses (i.e. 15 min/30 min/1 hr/2 hr/etc), stopping the doses when the symptoms abate. From 1 to 3 doses is usually all that is required.

Stop the remedy if there is no improvement after the third dose. Retake the case, using the Remedy Pictures to clarify your choice and to see if there is another suitable remedy. Choose carefully – although the remedies in this potency are safe, changing the remedies too often can confuse the symptom picture, making later or more expert diagnosis difficult.

Acute illness: Give 3–4 doses per day. Assess your choice of remedy after 3–4 doses by watching the body's signals; stop if better, continue if improving but lessen the frequency at this stage. Reassess if symptoms change or worsen.

For chronic illness: Suck one tablet or take 3–4 drops in a little water night and morning. Again, 1 to 3 doses is usually all that is required. In a chronic illness there may be no sign of improvement for up to ten days. Sometimes it can be seen much sooner than that. If symptoms worsen it is important to **stop taking the remedy**. Even if this is part of a general improvement the remedy has had its action and no more doses should be taken until the condition stabilizes again.

If there is no improvement after ten days, choose a different remedy, using the Remedy Pictures as a guide.

After a month, if the improvement has stopped, another prescription may be given. Retake the case, noting the symptoms anew to decide whether to repeat the same remedy or to give a new one. Once again, don't give your child too many remedies as it may confuse the symptom picture for the future. Be aware that a single dose can continue acting for months if not interfered with by further dosing.

EXTERNAL APPLICATIONS

Lotions and ointments made from homoeopathic remedies are available and can be applied to skin sores, bruises, wounds or painful areas as directed.

Do not use Arnica directly on an open wound as it stings.

NOTE

Some people continually fail to respond well to chosen remedies. The information under Resistance and Immunity (page 29) may be useful here, but constitutional treatment is more effectively undertaken by an experienced homoeopath or after detailed study of the Miasmic Remedies (which are not covered in this book).

You may find that one family member responds well to homoeopathics while another responds better to herbs or cell salts.

How to Use Cell Salts

READ THIS CHAPTER

Mineral salts are held together in the cellular tissues of the body in a delicate balance. They are vital to the proper growth and development of the body. An upset in the mineral balance heralds the beginning of illness.

Cell salts (also known as Tissue salts) are prepared into minute quantities on a lactose base, and are easily assimilated by the body. When correctly chosen, they aid in restoring equilibrium. For those on a dairy-free diet, cell salts are available in an alcohol base.

We have included a brief Remedy Picture (page 210) for each cell salt to help your selection.

Cell salts work well in a combination. However, they work best when alternated. Generally, no more than four is advisable either at any one time or (preferably) alternated at intervals throughout the day.

HOW CELL SALTS ARE TAKEN

Cell salts dissolve easily when sucked. For babies, crush the tablets between two clean teaspoons, drop water onto crushed tablets and feed on a teaspoon. For children, the tablets dissolve very quickly on the tongue.

In sudden, *acute* situations, 1–2 tablets can be taken every 10–15 minutes. For a baby, crush a tablet in a small $1/4$ cup of water and give a teaspoon dose at 10–15 minute intervals, increasing the time span between doses as severity of illness lessens. Discontinue when symptoms cease.

In *chronic*, longstanding situations, 1 tablet can be taken four times daily. If after seven days no improvement can be seen, it may be necessary to change or discontinue the cell salts. It is helpful to continue the cell salt(s) for several weeks after the illness has passed to ensure the original deficiency is overcome.

EXTERNAL APPLICATIONS

Cell salts may be crushed and mixed to a paste with a little water, then applied to affected skin areas.

RECOMMENDED CELL SALTS

There are twelve cell salts altogether:

Ferr Phos	Kali Mur
Nat Phos	Nat Sulph
Kali Phos	Kali Sulph
Calc Phos	Calc Sulph
Mag Phos	Calc Fluor
Nat Mur	Silica

How to Combine Remedies

READ THIS CHAPTER

Herbs and Homoeopathic Remedies

The mints, garlic, camphor, coffee, strongly aromatic inhalations and flavourings can antidote homoeopathic remedies so are best avoided when taking them.

Herbs are best taken at mealtimes and homoeopathic remedies a minimum of half an hour before or after taking food or drink. If you wish to use them both in the same day, it is wise to choose those remedies which relate to the same symptoms. Follow these rules, and herbs and homoeopathics will work harmoniously.

Herbs and Cell Salts

Choose cell salts and herbs which deal with the same symptoms. They can be taken together to repel invading toxins and strengthen the body during a crisis.

Cell Salts and Homoeopathic Remedies

A cell salt may help balance the metabolic processes by enhancing the use of a particular mineral while the homoeopathic remedy is working. In this situation you can combine them, taking the cell salt with meals and the homoeopathic remedy in between, but in the UK it is more common to stick with a single remedy.

Corresponding cell salt and homoeopathic remedies:

Calc Fluor   Silica, Kali Bich
Calc Phos   China, Ruta Grav, Calc Carb
Calc Sulph   Hepar Sulph, Silica
Ferr Phos   Aconite, Gelsemium
Kali Mur   Bryonia, Mercurius, Sulphur
Kali Phos   Rhus Tox, Phosphorus, Pulsatilla, Ignatia

Kali Sulph	Pulsatilla
Mag Phos	Belladonna, Colocynth
Nat Mur	Sepia, Sulphur, Phosphorus
Nat Phos	Calc Carb

Medical Drugs

Herbs, homoeopathics and cell salts work harmoniously with the body's natural healing activities, and can in many cases be helpful whilst under medication, by relieving side-effects of medical drugs without interfering with the main action of the drug. On the other hand, homoeopathic remedies may lose their effectiveness in the presence of particular drugs, e.g. steroids, cortisone, some laxatives, nose drops and liniments.

Resistance and Immunity

Constant exposure to processed and chemically treated food, frequent use of prescription drugs, environmental pollution and radiation all weaken the immune systems of our bodies. A weakened immune system contributes greatly to disease and poor recuperation. We can help our own and our children's immune systems by making appropriate changes to our life styles and by making good use of natural substances as described in this book.

DIET

1. Avoid foods which overload the system with waste products and rob the body of vital nutrients required to fight infection: chips, sweets, soft drinks, white flour and sugar products, fast foods, instant meals (frozen, canned or packaged), excess meat, chicken, excess dairy products and salty foods.

A note on dairy products and sugars:
Whilst dairy products unfortunately can create excess mucous and should be avoided if a child suffers from major catarrhal problems, they are very nourishing for a growing child. Pasteurized milk is devitalized and more mucous-forming than milk. However, unpasteurized is not recommended for children due to a risk of TB and is largely unavailable in the UK. If you want to give your child unpasteurized milk, the most easily digestible form is as follows: take $1/4$ to $1/2$ cup of milk, heat it to boiling point, add a pinch of spice such as cinnamon, cardamom or ginger, cool and sweeten with honey.

Yoghurt too has many qualities but can be quite heavy and hard to digest especially when taken with fruit (contrary to public opinion). The most digestible form of yoghurt is diluted 1:1 with water, the same spices and sweetener added as for milk above.

Sugars: Children need a certain amount of sugar for body-building. However, if it is over-refined, it leaches the minerals out of the body. Honey is a very concentrated sugar so use small amounts only. Other excellent sweeteners are: maple syrup, rice or barley malt and fruit concentrates.

2. Feed your children fresh food that has not been chemically treated, processed or devitalized with preservatives, colourings, or flavourings: fresh or dried fruit and vegetables; sprouted seeds and grains; pure diluted fruit juices; homemade cookies, cakes, pastries and breads made from wholegrain flours, honey and cold-pressed oils; grains, beans and unsalted nuts for protein and herbs and seeds for flavouring; eggs from free-range hens; and meat and chicken from organic farms.

BUILDING RESISTANCE

Herbs
A general herbal tonic and cleanser helps strengthen the immune system and neutralize toxins. The following herbs cleanse the lymphatic system and also act:

To purify the blood: Dandelion, Burdock, Echinacea
To detoxify the liver: Dandelion, Barberry
To stimulate circulation: Capsicum
To relieve lung congestion: Mullein
To help kidney action: Buchu, Uva Ursi
To cleanse lymphatic system: Calendula and all the above herbs
As antiseptic: Golden Seal, Myrrh
To help eliminate radiation and poisonous heavy metals: Irish Moss, Kelp
To aid digestion during the cleansing process: Rosemary, Rhubarb Root.

Choose your desired combination of herbs and make according to the instructions on page 16. Give daily for three weeks, rest for one week, repeat if necessary.

Homoeopathy
Homoeopathic Nosode remedies can help the body rebuild resistance and help strengthen the immune system against further attacks. They may be used:

1. If *during the actual illness* symptoms are especially trouble-some or if complications set in.
2. For failure to return to full health after a specific disease.
3. If a child *has never been well since being vaccinated* for the disease.

Take one dose (1 tablet or 2–3 drops of liquid) of the appropriate Nosode in the 30c potency. Give a second dose twenty-four hours later if there is no change.

Homoeopathic Nosodes
Chicken Pox: Varicella
Hepatitis: Hepatitis A or Hepatitis B
Infections (constant septic wounds): Staphylococcin/Streptococcin
Influenza: Influenzinum or Bacillinum
Measles: Morbillinum
Meningitis: Meningococcin
Mumps: Paratidinum
Polio: Polio
Pneumonia: Pneumococcin
German Measles: Rubella
Scarlet Fever: Scarletinum
Tetanus: Tetanotoxin
Tonsillitis: Streptococcin
Whooping Cough: Pertussin

IMMUNIZATION

Those who wish to be thoroughly informed about immunization need to read detailed and well-researched information from those pro-immunization (available through government and medical sources) and those anti-immunization (available through health clinics and some health shops). 'What Doctors Don't Tell You' gathers well-supported information on immunizations, their successes and failures. (WDDTY, 4 Wallace Road, London N1 2PG. Ph: (020) 7354-4592, Fax: (020) 7354-8907.)

Do You Plan To Vaccinate Your Child?
If so, we suggest you choose a remedy from the list below to counteract any ill effects of the vaccination and to remove the residual

toxins that may linger in the body and cause health problems now or later.

Homoeopathic remedies Give homoeopathic Thuja 12c the night before and the morning of the vaccination, and another dose immediately after. If the child seems unwell two weeks later, refer to Remedy Pictures (page 202) and choose the remedy which most closely matches your child's constitutional type.

Cell salts Alternatively, cell salts can be used. Kali Mur and Silica: one dose night and morning for seven days starting immediately after vaccination.

If, despite these precautions your child continues to suffer ill health after vaccination, the Nosode remedies may be given (see page 31). One dose of 30c potency is usually sufficient.

Occasionally a child will not respond to these remedies even when clearly selected. In these circumstances it will be necessary to consult an experienced homoeopath, who is trained to take a detailed case history and deal with the complex total symptom picture.

If You Don't Plan To Vaccinate Your Child
If this is you, you need to be aware that you are taking responsibility for your child's health. We advise that you maintain regular contact with an experienced homoeopath.

Caution
It is important to understand that homoeopathic remedies may fail to act if the inherent constitution of the child is weak or impaired in some way. This may or may not be apparent, so as a safeguard homoeopathy offers deep-acting remedies to strengthen a weak constitution. We recommend you seek expert homoeopathic advice or have a thorough knowledge of the Miasms before choosing to avoid vaccinations. (A Miasm is an inherited disease stigma which can be responsible for the apparent variations in health amongst different children despite similar socio-economic circumstances and dietary habits.)

Abscess

An abscess is a collection of pus formed when an infection caused by a germ is met by large numbers of white blood cells (to deal with the germs) and serum (to dilute and fight the toxins). This, together with increased blood supply to the area, causes redness, heat, swelling, pain and tenderness.

WHAT TO DO – External

Do not squeeze: This is very painful and can spread the infection into the system.

Herbs

Make a poultice using a double layer of clean fine gauze, large enough to cover the abscess. Between the layers place your choice from the following:

Comfrey Ointment or fresh crushed Comfrey leaves
Slippery Elm Powder (mixed to a paste with water)
Golden Seal Ointment
Teatree Oil used directly or diluted with Olive Oil

Place poultice over abscess. Cover with lint dressing or clean sheeting and secure with a plaster. Wear overnight and repeat daily. When the infection has cleared, use Hypercal Lotion for further healing.

Cell Salts

A solution of the appropriate remedy(s) from the list below can be used to bathe external parts by mixing three tablets with $1/2$ cup of reasonably hot water.

WHAT TO DO – Internal

Herbs

Usually, Vitamins A, B and C will be lacking. This deficiency can be corrected by purifying the blood and detoxifying the glands. Echinacea and Golden Seal are especially helpful in this; Dandelion, Dock, Comfrey or Poke Root may also be added.

Homoeopathic

Arsen Alb 30c: Burning pain, worse after midnight; better for heat applied to swelling.

Belladonna 30c: Sudden development, intense throbbing, bright red swelling. Use before pus has formed.

Hepar Sulph 30c: Sharp, sticking pain, beginning with chills, tender to touch.

Mercurius 30c: Great redness with stinging pain. Follows Belladonna after pus has formed.

Pyrogenium 30c: If abscess is swollen, discoloured and inflamed.

Anthracinum 30c: Black and blue abscess that looks decomposed.

Staphylococcin 30c: For recurrent abscesses once only.

Cell Salts

Ferr Phos: Redness, heat, pain and throbbing.

Kali Mur: For swelling, alternate with Ferr Phos throughout the day.

Silica: After swelling softens and pus begins to form. Warning: great care should be taken with using Silica. It can be very useful to treat abscesses around a foreign body and works to help the body to get rid of the foreign material – splinter, etc. However, it can also help the body get rid of dental caps and crowns, or screws and wires used to secure fractures.

Calc Sulph: If discharge continues too long.

Kali Phos: If discharge is putrid and foul-smelling.

HOW TO USE: HERBS, PAGE 16 | HOMOEOPATHICS, PAGE 20 | CELL SALTS, PAGE 25

AIDS/HIV

The following is a summary of information on AIDS as it relates to children.

Because new information on AIDS is constantly coming to light, it is important to keep up-to-date if you are concerned for any member of your family.

DESCRIPTION

Acquired Immune Deficiency Syndrome is caused by a virus now called HIV. Having AIDS means the immune system which usually fights disease slowly loses the ability to do so. The person becomes ill from some infection and, because of HIV, general health continues to deteriorate until a life-threatening illness cannot be fought off.

The disease can incubate for a period of three months, so some people can have the virus in their system and not feel sick or test positive. Even after a positive test or the incubation period is over they often remain well and healthy for many years without moving to full-blown AIDS. They can still infect others, however.

The symptoms of HIV are not listed here as they are similar to a number of ordinary childhood illnesses such as colds, bronchitis, influenza and diarrhoea. We believe that to associate such typical childhood symptoms with AIDS would cause undue anxiety. What distinguishes AIDS is the duration of such symptoms, their persistence, severity and their frequent co-existence with increasing general illness.

If you are very worried, there is a simple antibody test available which shows if someone has been in contact with HIV. However, anyone seeking this test is advised to first read the information about it and to seek counselling to explain the meaning of the test results.

HOW IS AIDS SPREAD?

HIV is difficult to catch. The virus is found in most body fluids – blood, semen, tears, breast milk and in blood in urine, faeces and saliva. It is spread when the virus comes into *direct* contact with the recipient's bloodstream, i.e. through cuts and abrasions.

Apart from the circumstances of sexual abuse, or contracting HIV at birth through infected parents, the possibility of a child catching HIV is still very low.

HOW AIDS IS NOT SPREAD

HIV has been found in dried material, but only in extremely small quantities. To date no known cases of HIV have been transmitted:

- By being near someone with AIDS/HIV
- To non-sexually involved people living with someone diagnosed as having AIDS/HIV
- To health workers through social contact alone or carrying out normal duties (however, there have been cases of health workers catching HIV, all of whom had open skin sores or needle stick injuries and didn't take the precautions listed below).
- Through casual contact with older children or living with children infected with AIDS/HIV
- Through casual contact like hugging, social kissing or using the same cutlery, dishes or washing facilities as someone with AIDS/HIV
- Through contact with toilet seats, door knobs, secondhand clothes, or anything else that has been touched by someone with AIDS/HIV.

It is extremely unlikely (although theoretically possible) that AIDS/HIV would be caught by biting or being bitten by someone who has AIDS/HIV. Swimming pools treated according to the advised requirements are reported as prohibiting the spread of AIDS/HIV.

PRECAUTIONS AGAINST HIV

When assisting someone who is bleeding, if you have reason for concern

1. Avoid contact with blood if you have open or unhealed cuts.
2. Use disposable gloves and afterwards wash thoroughly with

HOW TO USE: HERBS, PAGE 16 | HOMOEOPATHICS, PAGE 20 | CELL SALTS, PAGE 25

soap and water your hands, lower arms and any other part in contact with or splashed by blood.

3. Place any cotton wool, gauze, etc that has had contact with blood in a plastic bag and seal it for disposal.
4. Wipe down benches and other bloodied areas with cold or tepid water and then with household bleach freshly diluted 1:10 with water.
5. Wash with soap and water carpeted areas that have been splashed with blood.
6. Wash scissors or other instruments thoroughly in cold water to remove any blood, then sterilize by boiling in water for at least 10 minutes or by soaking for 30 minutes in household bleach diluted 1:10 with water.

Artificial Respiration Guards can be obtained for use in institutions and organizations. For accident victims *some* protection may be gained by using a hanky placed over the victim's mouth before beginning resuscitation.

Adolescents and young people need to know about HIV and the precautionary methods that help prevent the spread of all sexually transmitted diseases. If you have a teenager in your household, we recommend you obtain up-to-date, detailed information pamphlets from an AIDS clinic or your local Health Centre.

Playcentres, Kindergartens, Childcare Centres and Schools should already have received material from the Dept of Education discussing the above precautionary recommendations.

PREVENTION OF HIV

It is clear that some people are more susceptible than others to HIV and many lovers of people with HIV or recipients of contaminated blood have not developed and may never develop the disease. A strong immune system is maintained by good health. Poor nutrition, physical and psychological stress, heavy use of prescription or illegal drugs, repeated and poorly treated infections, constant exposure to environmental pollutants and/or adulterated food – all depress the immune system.

We can help our immune systems by being more aware of the above factors, making appropriate changes to our life styles and by making good use of the natural substances mentioned under Resistance and Immunity (see page 29).

Note: Although it is not yet adequately documented, there is evidence suggesting that the condition of HIV sufferers has improved after they have dealt with the above stress factors.

In recent years, with the combination of medical and natural approaches, there has been progress in dealing with AIDS/HIV.

HOW TO USE: HERBS, PAGE 16 | HOMOEOPATHICS, PAGE 20 | CELL SALTS, PAGE 25

Allergy

A hypersensitivity to certain foods, drugs, chemical additives or vapours, inhalants (dust, pollen, grasses, etc), insecticides, pillow and furniture stuffings and animal hairs (to name a few) is an indication of allergy. For allergic reactions to bee stings, see Bites and Stings.

DESCRIPTION

The most common symptom of allergy in children is hay fever. Allergy can also show itself in any of the following: hyperactivity, stress, depression, fear, anxiety, claustrophobia, bizarre behaviour, poor concentration and memory, bedwetting, vomiting, diarrhoea, asthma, skin rashes, sinus, bronchitis, eczema, hives, local swelling or blisters, itching burning eyes, earache and recurrent ear infections, reactions to insects bites, trembling, headaches, abdominal pain, joint aches, strong cravings, flatulence, cystitis.

Note: Faulty metabolism and digestion usually exist before an allergy occurs. Emotional disturbances may also be a factor.

Children usually crave or demand the food that they are allergic to. They will often throw tantrums when it is refused them. Once eaten, it will cause a temporary satisfaction as the withdrawal symptoms are relieved, but the metabolic system is placed under further strain.

TESTING FOR ALLERGIES
(Food, inhalants or skin irritants)

Method 1: Pulse acceleration test
1. Have child abstain from the suspected allergen for five days.
2. Take resting pulse (i.e. sit quietly for 10 minutes first). Write it down.
3. Expose your child to the suspected allergen. If a food, preferably eat only that food.
4. A minute after exposure take pulse again. Write it down.
5. Take pulse again 10 minutes later. Write it down.

6. Repeat 20 minutes later (i.e. 30 minutes after exposure). If the pulse has increased by 16 beats per minute or more, this substance is a stressor to your child.

Method 2: See a Touch for Health instructor
Any hypersensitivity is detected using a muscle testing process.

Method 3: Laboratory tests
Ask your local medical doctor about these.

Method 4: Allergy testing
A simple, non-invasive, painless and non-distressing test using a Vega machine. Appointments can usually be made at natural health clinics or shops.

WHAT TO DO

Allergies can be overcome without drugs. Carry out the allergy test Method 1 to determine what is an allergen for your child and choose any of these courses of action:

1. Exposure of the child (including the child in the womb) to many antibiotics or cortisones can produce overgrowth of the Candida Albicans organism. This can cause allergic reaction to yeast, marmite, yeast-based Vitamin Bs, wheat and sugars, especially refined carbohydrates such as cakes, biscuits and sweets. (See Thrush and deal with the Candida albicans infection as described there.)
    To replace the friendly bacteria in the small intestine, eat natural unsweetened yoghurt and/or take Lactobacillus Acidophilus tablets (available at most health shops).
2. Eliminate the allergen from your child's diet or environment. When the system has been under stress from an allergen, the problem becomes exacerbated and your child may test allergic to a great number of substances. Don't despair. Eliminate the suspect foods from your child's diet for 2–4 weeks. You will find that after a time you can safely reintroduce most of the offend-

HOW TO USE: HERBS, PAGE 16 | HOMOEOPATHICS, PAGE 20 | CELL SALTS, PAGE 25

ing foods – you will be left with the original allergen. However, it is important not to become paranoid, as it is not always possible to avoid allergens, or indeed identify them in the first place. Instead, work on regulating the digestive function by adding spices like nutmeg, cardamom, fennel, ginger to the daily diet.

3. Bach Flower Remedies are helpful for underlying emotional issues (available at most health shops).

4. Homoeopathy has a corresponding remedy for most common allergens. Seek expert homoeopathic advice from a registered homoeopath or from homoeopathic chemists listed on page 215.

5. See a Touch For Health instructor to rebalance the stress reaction to an allergen.

6. See an experienced natural health practitioner for difficult cases as constitutional issues must be dealt with.

Anaemia

A condition in which the circulating red blood cells are deficient in quantity or quality or both. It can be caused by: excessive blood loss (heavy periods, haemorrhage); deficiency in iron, folic acid, Vitamin B12 or thyroxine; chronic infection or inflammation (by snake venom, parasites, streptococci, bacteria, chemical agents); hereditary disorders; kidney disorders; malignancy or allergy.

DESCRIPTION

General tiredness, shortness of breath on exertion; giddiness; headache; pallor (especially of mucous membranes and palms of hands); palpitations; swollen ankles; indigestion; constipation; changeable mood patterns.

Note: Skin colour may be an unreliable test for anaemia because of variations in thickness and pigmentation of skin.

SEEK MEDICAL ADVICE

There are many types of anaemia, so blood and faeces tests are important to help establish the correct cause. Use the information below in addition to medical care.

WHAT TO DO

● Sunshine, open air and moderate exercise all help to improve the quality of the blood.

Foods
● Best foods are those rich in iron, B vitamins, manganese and hydrochloric acid: brewer's yeast, green leafy vegetables, sunflower seeds, sesame seeds, almonds, bananas, plums, strawberries, grapes, peaches, raisins, apples, apricots, figs, honey, lentils, goat's milk, buckwheat, rice, beans, safflower oil.
● Best juices are green vegetable, carrot and red beet, red grape, blackcurrant, prune and apricot. Take at least two glasses daily.

HOW TO USE: HERBS, PAGE 16 | HOMOEOPATHICS, PAGE 20 | CELL SALTS, PAGE 25

Herbs

For Iron: Yellow Dock, Golden Seal, Nettle, Raspberry, Rosehip, Basil.

For Vitamin B: Dandelion, Garlic, Kelp, Parsley, Chickweed, Hawthorn.

For Manganese: Black Walnut, Golden Seal, Watercress.

For Hydrochloric Acid: Safflowers.

To help build good blood: Red Clover, Echinacea, Myrrh, Liquorice, Barberry, Dandelion.

To help soothe intestinal lining in case of allergy: Comfrey, Slippery Elm.

To help increase red blood cells: Gentian, Thyme.

Homoeopathic

Alumina 30c: For anaemia at puberty with abnormal craving for indigestible substances, e.g. chalk, pencils.

Arsen Alb 30c: For pernicious anaemia; exhaustion, oedema, violent and irregular palpitations, craves acidic foods; extreme anxiety; irritable stomach, great thirst; looks weak and poorly.

Calc Carb 30c: For children disposed to obesity, catarrh and diarrhoea. Disgust for meat; craves sour, indigestible things; abdomen swollen; dizziness and palpitation on going upstairs; generally fearful.

China 30c: Anaemia due to fluid loss, haemorrhage, diarrhoea, too much menstrual flow; loss of vision, fainting, ringing in ears, pale, sallow complexion; sour belching, poor digestion, bloated abdomen; sensitive to draughts of air – better from fanning.

Ferr Met 30c: Bloated feeling followed by pale face and puffy extremities; mucous membranes are pale; easily exhausted, may vomit food after meals; constant chill; maybe fever in the afternoon.

Kali Carb 30c: Feels weak in heart region; backache; sweat; menstrual problems.

Nat Mur 30c: Good appetite but still thin and pale; throbbing headache, dyspnea (shortness of breath) worse from going upstairs; constipation, depression worse from being consoled; much fluttering and beating heart action; scanty menstruation.

Phosphorus 30c: Pernicious anaemia; very tired, rapid energy loss, puffy eyes.

Pulsatilla 30c: Antidotes ill-effects of too much iron. Chilly with gastric and menstrual disorders. Better in open air, dizzy on rising; no thirst; gentle, mild disposition.

Sepia 30c: Anaemia at puberty due to irregular menstruation; severe headache, sinking at pit of stomach; constipation with ineffectual urging and passing only wind and mucous.

Cell Salts

Alternate Ferr Phos and Calc Phos twice weekly each for six months if symptoms suit.

Calc Phos (helps to supply new blood cells): Face pale, greenish caused by poor nutrition; thin, delicate pale infants; anaemia after exhausting diseases. Waxy skin, headache, ringing ears, dizziness, cold extremities, heavy menstruation.

Ferr Phos: Follows Calc Phos as improvement sets in. Use for deficiency in haemoglobin. Pale face, flushes easily, pale lips; tendency to coughs and headaches. Ferr Phos is the normal constituent of tissues and is more easily assimilated than inorganic iron tonics.

Nat Mur: For young girls with dirty complexion; dry, scaly skin, constipation with very dry stools; palpitations; melancholy with bad dreams, backache, chills, fevers and perspiration.

Silica: For longstanding signs of anaemia in poorly nourished children.

HOW TO USE: HERBS, PAGE 16 | HOMOEOPATHICS, PAGE 20 | CELL SALTS, PAGE 25

Anxiety

This section includes behavioural disorders and learning difficulties.

Anxiety is an exaggerated or inappropriate response to stress. It is characterized by feelings of anticipation, uneasiness, apprehension or alarm often unrelated to anything or anyone in particular.

Note: In some situations anxiety can act as a positive device warning us against danger. Our concern here is with overwhelming or frequently recurring anxiety.

Anxiety can be caused by: emotionally disturbing experiences, bad frights, encounters with hostile or disagreeable people; domestic strife; school phobias; lack of self-confidence; overwork; persistently poor communication with parents, family, school teachers or peers; feelings of being unloved and unwanted (e.g. after new brother or sister or step parent). Can also be caused by psychological imbalances due to dietary imbalances, e.g. lack of calcium; overdose of sugars or caffeine products or can be part of a depressive illness.

DESCRIPTION

Physical symptoms may be palpitations, tremors, diarrhoea, urinary frequency, headache, hyperventilation, stomach ache, insomnia, nervousness, trembling.

Alternatively, the child may manifest undesirable behavioural patterns such as: nail biting, temper tantrums, stealing, truancy, unmanageability, learning difficulties, dyslexia.

Note: While occasional incidents like these can be considered 'normal' during a child's development, habitual, compulsive or disabling behaviour patterns need to be addressed.

WHAT TO DO

Rather than label these symptoms as psychoneuroses or personality disturbances, we look upon them as indications of a lack of balance or harmony between the body, mind and emotions. While some children will respond favourably to the homoeopathic approach, others may require Bach Flower Remedies to calm their emotions, or will benefit from nutritional improvements, especially in the form of herbs, and the removal of junk foods from the diet. If you wish to follow these courses of action, seek further advice from a homoeopath, natural health practitioner, or the books on Bach Flowers (available in most health shops).

There are also many techniques available to help us verbalize thoughts and feelings to become aware of how stress and anxiety affect ourselves and our children. We can help by supporting and reassuring the child, and by making an effort to understand what they are going through.

Sometimes it is necessary to balance the left and right hemispheres of the brain. To this end, there are many safe techniques available which teach how to balance mind, body and emotions. These include One Brain, Touch for Health, Counselling, NLP Psychotherapy and so on.

Herbs
The following combination taken daily for several months can help to calm the nerves: Valerian, Lavender, Passionflower, Vervain, Melissa and/or Rosemary.

Homoeopathic
Aconite 30c: For acute anxiety, extreme impatience, intolerance of pain, music, least noise; horrible fears; usually triggered by acute clearcut cause (e.g. fright). Fear of crowds and open spaces.

Argent Nit 30c: Dreadful anticipation, impulsive, nervous; bites nails, tearful and apprehensive before ordeal of any kind; fear of heights, going to school, closed spaces, water, exams, stage-fright.

Arnica 30c: Where there is a history of injury or fright; great fear with inconsolable anxiety and restlessness.

Arsen Alb 30c: Sensitive to disorder and confusion; can't sleep in a messy room; imagines burglars; dreams of darkness, fire and danger. Changes place continually. Fears being alone.

Arum Triph 30c: Bites nails, picks at lips and nose, restless and irritable.

HOW TO USE: HERBS, PAGE 16 | HOMOEOPATHICS, PAGE 20 | CELL SALTS, PAGE 25

Baryta Carb 30c: Child is bashful, slow developer, acts stupid; doesn't want to play, prefers to sit idly in a corner.

Belladonna 30c: Imaginary fears, wants to run away. Delirious; violent impulses. Bed wetting.

Borax 30c: Dread of downward motion. Anxious and afraid of falling.

Calc Carb 30c: Night terrors; great anxiety and restlessness; visions of faces and people on closing eyes; school phobias; self-willed; insecure; always putting strange things into mouth, e.g. chalk, pencils.

Chamomilla 30c: Temper tantrums, whining, everything wrong, little things annoy; likes to be carried; can't bear pain; stubborn and obstinate.

Gelsemium 30c: Depressed, timid, anxious, tired, lazy, sluggish, worse after a bout of influenza; insecure, fear of failing, apprehension before an ordeal; tremulous and shaky.

Ignatia 30c: Stammering; feels effect of sudden shock or stress; depressed and irritable; bottles things up; dwells on problems in secret; bears grudges; sighs frequently; cannot bear pain or criticism.

Kali Phos 30c: Doesn't like meeting people; jumpy and nervous at the slightest thing; everything seems too much trouble.

Nux Vomica 30c: Frustrated, quarrelsome, critical, hypersensitive, aggressive.

Pulsatilla 30c: Emotionally upset and anxious, tearful and touchy, worse from bad news.

Tuberculinum 30c: Child afraid of animals, especially dogs; uses foul language, curses and swears; sensitive and dissatisfied; excited one minute, tearful the next.

Veratrum Album 30c: Tells lies, tears things, swears, inclined to run away; refuses to talk; sings, whistles, laughs or acts insane.

Cell Salts

Kali Phos: Most important remedy – depressed; irritable, bad-tempered; sleep-walking, starts talking, wakes at slightest sound; timid, blushing, starts at sudden noise; exhausted from overwork; phobias, hallucinations, raving.

Nat Mur: Sad, apprehensive, negative thinker; hates being consoled, avoids company, easily annoyed; palpitations.

Herbs

Calamus Root: helps improve intelligence, concentration and will-power.

Gotu Kola: helps improve mental power, purifies the blood, calms the emotions.

SLOW DEVELOPMENT

Occasionally the above disorders can be due to a lesion of the central nervous system caused by heredity, trauma or environmental causes (e.g. meningitis, birth injury, malformation, deprivation of social stimuli such as deaf mutes).

These children will be immature and slow to develop, they may appear to lack intelligence and mental control, physical control or have some form of spasticity or deformity. One Brain and Touch for Health techniques will be of the utmost benefit (see a Touch for Health or One Brain instructor) and it is wise to combine these techniques with the appropriate remedies listed below.

Homoeopathic

Arnica 30c: Where a history of trauma has blocked the child's progress to maturity.

Baryta Carb 30c: For very slow psychological maturity.

Calc Carb 30c: Usually placid and obstinate, immature, withdrawn, exhausted, all life seems an effort.

Silica 30c: Refined and senstitive, stunted growth physically and mentally, leaving the child weak and vulnerable with profuse sweating and no physical energy.

Thyroidinum 30c: For stunted physical growth and very sluggish metabolism.

Tuberculinum 30c: Helps stimulate psychological maturity, especially where child is anxious and restless.

HOW TO USE: HERBS, PAGE 16 | HOMOEOPATHICS, PAGE 20 | CELL SALTS, PAGE 25

Asthma

A disorder of the bronchial tubes (air tubes). Asthma is considered an allergic reaction but infections, psychological and emotional factors are frequently involved as well. The bronchial muscles go into spasm and there is increased mucous production by the mucous glands. This narrowing of the air passages, congested with mucous, makes breathing difficult. Air is easier to draw in than out and the air trapped in the lungs makes oxygenation more difficult. If the disease starts in early childhood, there is a 20–30 per cent chance of spontaneous recovery.

DESCRIPTION

Alarming difficulty in breathing (especially exhaling), creating a musical wheeze from deep in the lungs. There may be a cough. The skin may have a bluish tinge. Attacks are most often at night, or early morning, and may last several hours or days.

SEEK MEDICAL ATTENTION

Always seek urgent medical attention for an acute asthma attack. Correctly used natural remedies can also offer significant help to asthma sufferers.

WHAT TO DO – Acute Attack

- If your child is susceptible to asthma attacks, have something already prepared.
- There are immediate measures that you may find helpful: Place child in the position which makes breathing easiest – usually upright with back straight, leaning slightly forward. Your instinct may be to hold him tightly out of fear. Although it is important to reassure the child, give him breathing space, and remain calm yourself with Rescue Remedy or Aconite at 15-minute intervals. Seek urgent medical attention.

Herbs

Tea: Make a tea from your choice of the following herbs and have the child sip this frequently throughout the acute period.

To help relieve bronchial tension: Lobelia Tincture (1 drop for each year of child's age – some children react strongly to this herb so it is wise to begin with a low dose).

To reduce the mucous build-up: Lungwort, Mullein, Elecampane or Hops.

To help soothe the lungs: Comfrey, Slippery Elm or Marshmallow.

To help relieve spasms and calm the nerves: Lemon, Lavender or Aniseed (can be obtained in oil form and added to tea in doses of 1 drop).

Inhalation: Mix Lavender (3 drops), Eucalyptus (2 drops) and Thyme (1 drop) Oils with hot water in a bowl and have child breathe this in deeply to help ease the congestion and tightness. (This process is more effective with towel over head and bowl to retain steam.)

Massage: The above Oils mixed with Olive or Almond Oil are soothing when rubbed onto the chest and spinal areas.

Homoeopathic

Antim Tart 30c: For great rattling of mucous with pounding chest, worse lying down; child must sit up to breathe more easily.

Arsen Alb 30c: Worse 1–2 am, cold air, movement or lying down. Burning feeling in chest, rapid heart beat, great exhaustion accompanies the attack; better from bending forward, warmth and hot drinks.

Ipecac 30c: May result from inhaling dust. Loose rattling cough, with gagging or vomiting but mucous does not come up. Great weight and anxiety in chest. Worse from motion.

Kali Bich 30c: Stringy, yellow mucous, worse morning and 2–3 am, child feels better by bending forward and coughing up mucous.

Nat Sulph 30c: Asthma comes on with damp weather. Rattling in chest, worse 4 am, child must hold chest. Every cold brings on asthma.

HOW TO USE: HERBS, PAGE 16 | HOMOEOPATHICS, PAGE 20 | CELL SALTS, PAGE 25

Nux Vomica 30c: Comes on after stomach upsets with belching and nausea. Worse in the morning and on a full stomach. Must loosen clothing.

Cell Salts

Alternate Ferr Phos, Kali Phos and Mag Phos at 10-minute intervals. If one appears to be more effective than the others, then you may give more of it.

To build resistance: Choose one or more of the following and have child take them twice daily for at least two weeks.

Nat Sulph: Greenish expectoration.

Calc Phos: Clear, tough expectoration.

Silica: Hay asthma, starts as itching and tingling in nose with discharge.

WHAT TO DO – Long-Term Approach

During absence of attack, treatment must be undertaken to strengthen the lungs, relieve mucous congestion and build up the body's vital force so that it can withstand the next attack more readily.

- In some cases, misalignment of the spine can be a major contributing factor as some dorsal nerves link directly with the lungs. Suspect this if the shoulder blades poke out abnormally, or if child has had a bad fall in the past. If necessary, see an osteopath or chiropractor about this.
- Always suspect allergies as potential causes of an asthmatic condition, either in the form of food or inhalants. See Allergy on how to deal with this. Consider temperature and climate in your region as these may aggravate the situation.
- If the child develops cold, bronchitis and influenza, use treatment advised under these headings in this book to ward off possible attack.
- Check emotional stress. This can be a major contributing factor, so find someone who knows about Bach Flowers to help out. Books on Bach Flowers are available at most health shops.
- Take herbs rich in Vitamins A, C and E such as: Coltsfoot, Comfrey, Burdock, Yellow Dock, Oats, Gentian and Elecampane.

- Keep the child's stress down to a minimum. These children are usually very sensitive to *your* stress levels so keep yourself relaxed also. Relaxing herbs are Chamomile, Passionflower, Mistletoe, Lavender or Lemon.
- If there is a history of infections, add Golden Seal, Southernwood and Poke Root to the herbal combination. If the child has a tendency to constipation, add Senna or Rhubarb Root.

If the child is on medication you should not stop it immediately but seek advice.

HOW TO USE: HERBS, PAGE 16 | HOMOEOPATHICS, PAGE 20 | CELL SALTS, PAGE 25

Babies and Nursing Mothers

BABIES

Herbs

The breastfeeding mother can drink herbal tea and the benefits of the herb will be passed on to the baby through the milk.

Alternatively, make a mild infusion of $1/4$ to $1/2$ tsp of dried herbs per cup of boiling water and give small amounts to baby on a teaspoon.

Using these guidelines, see individual headings for: Constipation, Diarrhoea, Sleep, Teeth, and Nappy Rash.

Cradle Cap: Rub Wheatgerm Oil, Apricot Kernel Oil or Castor Oil onto scalp daily.

Infected Umbilical Cord: Apply a few drops of Myrrh or Propolis Tincture after bathing and several times throughout the day.

Colic: Make mild infusion of Catnip, Chamomile, Dill, Fennel or Ginger. Give in teaspoonful doses when rested.

Homoeopathic

Homoeopathic remedies are rapid in action and are taken in minute amounts. They are available mostly in tablets, so crush them or dissolve in water, giving one teaspoon to one dose. See under individual headings for: Constipation, Diarrhoea, Sleep, Teeth, Nappy Rash.

Colic

Bryonia 30c: Irritable from least movement; can't stand to be soothed.

Chamomilla 30c: Often has one red cheek and other pale. Cranky and impossible.

Colocynth 30c: Child doubles up with pain. Better from firm pressure on abdomen.

Mag Phos 30c: Colic better from warmth and gentle pressure on abdomen.

Difficult birth or shock after an easy birth can sometimes cause the body great psychological stress which shows in difficult breathing, colour changes, limp limbs, sucking difficulty, etc. (Although births are attended by a doctor/midwife, the following remedies can be used.)

Arnica 30c: For shock, bruising, limp limbs, difficult sucking. (Rescue Remedy can also be used for shock.)

Aconite 30c: Purple-coloured face, shocked, frightened or anxious.

Antim Tart 30c: Difficulty in breathing due to pressure and delay of difficult birth. Rattling in throat.

Carbo Veg 30c: For pale, cold, limp limbs.

Laurocerasus 30c: Breathless and blue, failing pulse. No rattle in throat.

Feeding problems

Aethusa 30c: Milk is vomited in large oily curds as soon as swallowed. Infant is exhausted afterwards.

Calc Carb 30c: Hungry but dislikes the taste of the milk; these infants have large heads, large open fontanelles and a chalky colouring.

Calc Phos 30c: Infant wants to nurse constantly but vomits and develops diarrhoea easily.

Mag Carb 30c: Colic. Intolerant of milk. Infant easily develops constipation.

Nat Carb 30c: Infant dislikes milk which can cause thrush or diarrhoea; abdomen becomes hard, bloated and swollen, loud rumblings and pain.

Nux Vomica 30c: Blocked nose interferes with breastfeeding. Delayed meconium. Child is restless and uneasy. Hiccoughs.

Tuberculinum 30c: Markedly worse from milk. Easy vomiting of milk. Very irritable.

Infantile jaundice

Chelidonium or China 30c.

Lycopodium 30c

Sulph 30c

Nat Sulph 30c

Wheatgerm Oil (2–3 drops in the mouth daily) can also help.

Skin problems can appear within the first few days.

HOW TO USE: HERBS, PAGE 16 | HOMOEOPATHICS, PAGE 20 | CELL SALTS, PAGE 25

Arnica Tincture: Apply externally to any bruised skin – avoid eyes
and broken skin.
Arnica 30c: For bruising.
Calc Phos 30c: Bleeding from the navel.
Calc Fluor 30c: Birth marks. This can also be taken as cell salt (6x).
Thuja Tincture can also be applied to affected skin area.
Medorrhinum 30c: For constipation with fiery, red rash around anus
and severe nappy rash.
Phosphorus 30c: Moisture oozing from navel.
Sulphur 30c: Raw, chafed skin around anus.

Sore eyes
Aconite 30c: Red, inflamed, watering eyes.
Belladonna 30c: Red, swollen and dry eyes. Worse from light.
Chamomilla 30c: Swollen and gummed-up eyelids. Often one red
cheek.
Pulsatilla 30c: Swollen eyes with white or creamy, bland discharge.
Mercurius 30c: Red eyes and lids with yellowish discharge.
Urine retention during first eighteen hours: Aconite 30c.

MOTHERS

Herbs
To increase milk supply: Aniseed, Blessed Thistle, Caraway,
Fennel, Fenugreek, Rue, Vervain and/or Nettle.
To decrease milk supply: Sage, parsley.
To regulate milk supply and aid lactation in general: Black Cohosh,
Ginger, Liquorice, Marshmallow, Poke Weed, Yarrow.
To combat engorgement and breast infection, Vitamin C-rich herbs:
Cayenne, Blessed Thistle, Poke Root, Echinacea. Ginger poul-
tice applied externally. Make hot compresses from Comfrey
leaves, Cabbage leaves, Mullein or Lobelia.
For cracked nipples: Poke Root poultice. Rub with Wheatgerm Oil.

Homoeopathic remedies
Shock and Bruising: Arnica 30c immediately after birth.
Pain of Episiotomy: Hypericum or Staphysagria 30c.
After-pains: Mag Phos or Cimicifuga Racemosa 30c.
Exhaustion: China 30c or Cocculus 30c.

Feeding Problems

Belladonna 30c: Breasts swollen, congested, hard and hot with red streaks. Very tender. Abscess.

Bryonia 30c: Painful breast engorgement, worse from any movement, better from pressure. Mastitis.

Chamomilla 30c: Cracked nipples, cries out in pain, very irritable and emotional. Suppressed milk due to particular event.

Lac Deflor 30c: Insufficient milk.

Lycopodium 30c: Sore, bleeding and cracked nipples.

Nat Sulph 30c: Too much milk.

Petroleum 30c: Itchy, mealy covering of nipples.

Phytolacca 30c: Nipples sore with intense suffering on suckling which radiates all over body. Abscess.

Pulsatilla 30c: Too much or thin, watery milk. Pains extend to chest, neck and down back. Suppression of milk due to shock or particular event. Insufficient milk. Also useful to reduce flow during weaning.

Sepia 30c: Deep, sore cracks across crown of nipple. Aversion to breast feeding.

Sulphur 30c: Nipple smarts, burns and chaps badly; looks unclean.

Urtica Urens 30c: Insufficient milk. Swollen breast.

Post-Partum Depression

Ignatia 30c: Tearful and sighing a great deal.

Kali Carb 30c: Weak, irritable, tired, not usual self.

Nat Mur 30c: Wants to be alone; hides feelings but easily tearful; worse when consoled.

HOW TO USE: HERBS, PAGE 16 | HOMOEOPATHICS, PAGE 20 | CELL SALTS, PAGE 25

Bites and Stings

Dog Bites

If skin is not broken, wash thoroughly with Hypercal Lotion (10 drops to $1/2$ glass water) several times over the next few days and watch for any worsening of condition. It is vital to have an anti-tetanus injection.

If skin is broken, clean it as above, and take internally: Belladonna 30c once daily for seven days, then once weekly for six weeks. Follow-up remedy can be selected from the list below.

Jellyfish

Apis 30c: Give at 15-minutes intervals 4–5 times.
Medusa 30c: If skin problems linger despite taking Apis.

Bees, Wasps

A bee sting contains muscles that continue to pump poison into the skin so the first priority is to remove the sting quickly. Be sure to flick sideways with the fingernail. Make sure you do not press the bag as more poison will be pushed in.

A wasp has distinct yellow and black stripes and retains its sting.

Allergic reaction: Rapid, gross swelling starting at point of sting and spreading. Child often shows stress symptoms. Give Histamine 30c; Apis 30c.

SEEK MEDICAL ADVICE

If sting is on head or neck, or if sting is causing breathing difficulty. (Both orthodox and homoeopathic practitioners offer a course of treatment to counteract allergic reactions.)

Fleas and Mosquitoes

The occasional flea or mosquito bite can be alleviated with a dab of Aloe Vera Gel or the herbs or homoeopathics recommended below. However, numerous bites can cause great itching, irritation and even infected skin.

- Homoeopathic Ledum 6X once daily can act as a repellent during the mosquito season.
- When a house has been infested with fleas, Epsom Salts sprinkled or Pennyroyal Oil sprayed on the beds and floor will help prevent reinfestation.

WHAT TO DO

The following advice applies to skin affections from any of the above.

Herbs

Apply directly to bite or sting for relief:

- Crushed leaves of Plantain, Dock, Mint, Marigold, Summer Savory, Basil
- Oils of Teatree, Sage, or Lavender
- Aloe Vera Gel or Comfrey Ointment.

Homoeopathic

Apis 30c: For bites and stings that burn and sting, for swelling about the throat and maybe the entire body; better from cold water, worse from heat, touch or pressure.

Culex 30c: For lingering skin problems after mosquito bites.

Hepar Sulph 30c: Where skin becomes infected and sensitive to touch and cold.

Histamine 30c: For gross swellings or allergic reactions. Can be taken simultaneously with one of the other remedies.

Ledum 30c: For puncture wounds caused by bees, wasps, mosquitoes, or rats, where sensations are tingling, pricking, gnawing, itching. Worse from heat, movement and scratching.

Pulex 30c: For lingering skin problems after flea bites.

Rhus Tox 30c: For itching and swelling which is better from warm applications. Use this remedy when there is no improvement from Urtica Urens or Ledum. Do not use before or after Apis.

Urtica Urens 30c: For pain, swelling and intolerable itching of bee stings. There may be puffiness, intense burning, redness and stinging worse on hands and feet. This can be taken internally,

HOW TO USE: HERBS, PAGE 16 | HOMOEOPATHICS, PAGE 20 | CELL SALTS, PAGE 25

but also is safe to apply the tincture at 5-minute intervals on a compress when the face or eyelid are affected.

External applications: Tinctures of Arnica, Urtica Urens, Plantago or Ledum can be applied together or separately to the bites or stings.

Cell Salts

Nat Mur: First remedy for bites and stings, relieves pain, can be used internally or externally.

Kali Phos: If antiseptic is needed.

Kali Mur: Follows Nat Mur for subsequent swelling.

Blisters

A raised fluid-filled bubble of skin caused by local serum build-up under the skin in response to burns (see Burns) or local irritation. Single blisters are not serious, but once opened are liable to infection.

WHAT TO DO

For any blister that starts to fester, **seek medical advice**.

For single blisters caused by local irritation:

- Use a pre-packed sterile needle. Slanting the needle along the skin, slide it into the side of the blister to release the fluid serum. Soak up the fluid with cotton wool soaked in Hypercal solution. However, there is an argument that piercing the blister encourages infection.
- Choose *one* of the following procedures:
  Cover with Calendula Cream and plaster.
  Dab with cotton wool soaked in Hypercal solution and cover
    with gauze firmly secured with tape or plaster.
  Dab with Apricot Oil mixed with a little Lavender Oil.

HOW TO USE: HERBS, PAGE 16 | HOMOEOPATHICS, PAGE 20 | CELL SALTS, PAGE 25

Boils

An infection that forms a sac of pus under the skin in a hair follicle, a pore in the skin, or a puncture wound.

DESCRIPTION

Starts as an itchy red swelling on the skin. The inflammation in a confined space becomes very painful and the swelling increases. A hard core of dead tissue then forms in the centre of fluid pus. Can form in groups. Boils can cause swollen glands and fever.

WHAT TO DO – External

Do not squeeze. This is very painful and can spread the infection into the system.

Make a poultice using a piece of double-layered gauze, large enough to cover the boil, and placing in it your choice of the following:

Comfrey Ointment or fresh crushed Comfrey leaves
Slippery Elm Powder mixed to a paste with water
Hypercal Lotion (10 drops to $1/2$ glass water) – dressing can be moistened with this mixture.
Golden Seal Ointment

Place poultice over boil, cover with lint dressing or clean sheeting and secure with tape or plaster. Wear overnight and repeat daily until boil is cleaned. When boil softens, core comes away with the dressing. Now clean with Hypercal for antiseptic and to help avoid scarring.

For bathing, make a solution of the appropriate cell salt remedy – crush 3 tablets to $1/2$ cup of water.

INTERNAL APPROACH

Herbs
Cleanse the system internally with Vitamin A and C-rich herbs such as: Yellow Dock, Burdock, Poke Root, Queens Delight and/or Echinacea. Golden Seal is also useful for its antiseptic properties.

Homoeopathic

Anthracinum 30c: Black and blue sores that decompose quickly and have black centres.

Arnica 30c: Crops of small boils all over the body.

Pyrogenium 30c: Swollen, inflamed and discoloured-looking boils. Better from heat.

Rhus Tox 30c: Red, swollen and itchy; accompanied by swollen glands.

Silica 30c: Boils discharge their pus and do not heal readily.

Staphylococcin 30c: For recurring boils.

Cell Salts

Ferr Phos: Redness, heat, pain and throbbing.

Kali Mur: For swelling, alternate this with Ferr Phos.

Silica: After swelling softens, and pus begins to form. Also use after boil has broken.

Calc Sulph: If discharge continues too long.

Kali Phos: If discharge looks and smells foul.

LONG-TERM APPROACH

Boils indicate an underlying toxic condition of the blood. Recurring boils may be a symptom of diabetes or due to fatigue, excess consumption of refined foods (white flour, sugar products etc), poor elimination, faulty hygiene, or stress. Take steps to deal with these factors. Cleanse the system with the herbs listed above made into a tea and taken daily for one month. Also Staphylococcin 30c may be taken once only for recurring boils.

SEEK MEDICAL ADVICE

If inflammation continues and spreads.

HOW TO USE: HERBS, PAGE 16 | HOMOEOPATHICS, PAGE 20 | CELL SALTS, PAGE 25

Bronchitis

Acute inflammation of the bronchial tubes (air passages of the lungs) which begins as an upper respiratory tract infection.

DESCRIPTION

Fever, hacking cough, sore throat; may be difficult breathing; pain in lungs or back, rattling sound in chest.

WHAT TO DO

Best foods are fresh fruits and vegetables. Avoid dairy products, sweets and wheat products as these can create excess mucous.

Herbs

Make a tea, combining your choice of the following:

> *To loosen and help remove phlegm:* Comfrey, Elecampane, Mullein or Hyssop.
>
> *To soothe the inflamed surfaces:* Liquorice, Marshmallow or Slippery Elm.
>
> *For fever:* Lemon Balm, Elder Flower or Boneset.
>
> *To purify the blood:* Red Clover, Thyme or Poke Root.

Inhalation: Two drops of Thyme, Lemon and/or Peppermint Oils can be added to steaming water. Cover head and bowl with towel and breathe in the steam to clear the air passages and loosen mucous.

Chest rub: Two drops Thyme, Teatree and/or Clove Oil can be mixed with $1/2$ cup of Olive or Soya Oil and rubbed on chest several times daily.

Bath: The same oils can be added to bath water (foot bath is beneficial).

Homoeopathic

Aconite 30c: Hoarse, dry cough; frequent sneezing; loud breathing; short of breath with anxiety and restless sleep. Use at first stage of illness and fever.

Antim Tart 30c: Rattling chest but very little mucous is raised. Child may be wheezing, drowsy, and feels worse from drinking milk or lying down. Must sit up to breathe.

Bryonia 30c: Dry cough, needs to breathe deeply, worse from motion, better whilst resting; stitching pain in sides of chest. Must sit up to cough.

Hepar Sulph 30c: Loose, rattling moist cough, hoarse voice, yellow expectoration. Worse from cold, touch or at least uncovering.

Kali Bich 30c: Tough mucous, thick and stringy, difficult to raise. Worse in morning, worse eating. Often accompanied by swollen glands.

Phosphorus 30c: Tickling cough; hot, tight chest; trembling during cough; pain as if something were torn loose in chest; worse from talking or laughing, cold air, touch, exertion. Better from dark and sleep. Use Phosphorus also for head colds that tend to go to the chest, and for lingering cases.

Pulsatilla 30c: Loose, thick, yellow-green mucous may be coughed up. Cough tends to be dry in the evenings and loose in the morning. Pressure and soreness of chest.

Cell Salts

Ferr Phos: For first stage with heat, fever, cough with no mucous. Then when cough loosens alternate with Kali Mur.

Kali Mur: Thick, white and loose mucous may be coughed up.

Kali Sulph: Copious discharge of yellow, green mucous. Continue to alternate this with Ferr Phos while there is a fever.

Silica: Thick, yellow, heavy mucous is coughed up. Worse from cold drinks, better from warm drinks.

CHRONIC BRONCHITIS

Is indicated where there are repeated attacks.

- Use the above herbs regularly for 2 or 3 weeks. These herbs are rich in Vitamin A and are much needed to help strengthen the lungs.

HOW TO USE: HERBS, PAGE 16 | HOMOEOPATHICS, PAGE 20 | CELL SALTS, PAGE 25

- Also use the appropriate cell salt twice daily for a couple of weeks only but include Ferr Phos to oxygenate the lungs.
- Tuberculinum 30c: This is useful when response to homoeopathic treatment is poor. Thick, easy expectoration. Craves cold air. Short of breath.

Make sure the child is not exposed to cigarette smoke (yours or anyone else's). This can be as bad for her as if she were smoking herself.

Bruises

Mechanical damage to the blood vessels or muscles beneath the skin without breaking skin surface. When damage is done to deeper layers without breaking the skin, this is considered a contused wound (see Wounds).

WHAT TO DO

Herbs

Make poultice using clean double-layered gauze large enough to cover bruised area. Place in it any of the following:

Comfrey Ointment or fresh crushed Comfrey leaves.
Arnica Ointment.
Slippery Elm Powder mixed to a paste with a little water.

Place poultice against bruised area, place second, larger piece of lint or sheeting, and secure with tape or plaster.

Homoeopathic

Arnica 30c: Initially for all bruising.
Hypericum 30c: Nerve or spinal bruises. Very painful injuries. Crush injuries.
Rhus Tox 30c: Damage to muscle, ligaments or tendons.
Ruta Grav 30c: Bone and eye injuries.

External application: Moistened, crushed tablets can also be applied with lint dressing and bandage.

HOW TO USE: HERBS, PAGE 16 | HOMOEOPATHICS, PAGE 20 | CELL SALTS, PAGE 25

Burns

Damage to body tissues caused by exposure to excess heat. This may be due to fire, flame, electric current, sun rays, steam, abrasions, caustic substances, dry ice, boiling liquid, tar or oil, friction.

Dangers from burns are: circulatory collapse from pain; shock; serum loss; fluid seeping out from the burned surface can deplete the body of vital proteins, salt and water; and infection.

DESCRIPTION

Major Burns

- More than ten per cent of the body surface is burned. The larger the area burned the greater the effect on the circulation and the more seriously ill the child will be.
- Destruction of full thickness of the skin. Fat and muscles are burned. Burns have a yellow-white appearance. The area is often not painful as nerve endings are destroyed.
- All burns around joints should also be treated as major.

Minor Burns

Damage to outer skin layers only. Red and painful. Maybe blisters.

WHAT TO DO

1. *For major burns – ring ambulance or doctor immediately.*
2. Run cold water gently over burned area for at least ten minutes or until burning sensation ceases. Continue further procedures as necessary – see below.
3. Give Arnica 30c or Rescue Remedy (4 drops on tongue).
4. Lay child down, cover larger burns with clean sheeting (nappy or pillowcase will do).
5. Keep child warm but do not overheat.
6. Give frequent small drinks of water (unless unconscious). Rescue Remedy or Arnica (4 drops to $1/2$ glass of water) can be added to this or placed directly on to tongue or lips.
7. Reassure frequently.

Scalding Clothes: If clothes hold scalding or corrosive liquid do not remove any clothing that is already stuck to the skin and pulling skin away; nor if skin is black and sticky. Instead, keep skin and clothes soaking and ring for doctor and ambulance immediately.

Acid Burns: Bathe burn in mixture of bicarbonate of soda (baking soda) and water (2 tsp to 1 litre or approximately 1 packet to a bath for larger burns).

Burns from Caustic Soda, Ammonia or Lime: Immediately put in water, then as soon as possible bathe burn in equal parts vinegar (or lemon juice) and water.

If Clothes Catch Fire: Smother flames by wrapping rug, blanket or coat around child. Roll on ground to help put out flames: douse smouldering clothes and child with water.

Burns from Electric Current: After electric shock, child will either be thrown clear or go into muscle spasm and may remain attached to source.

Do not endanger yourself. Cut off current at main or push child off using *wooden* handled broom. Check breathing. Burns will show only at entry and exit points of current and may appear minor. Electric current causes damage along the whole length of the path travelled, internal and external.

Always seek medical help.

Sunburn: If sun exposure has caused burning, use procedures as indicated below to help prevent potential skin problems.

IMPORTANT

- DO NOT endanger yourself
- DO NOT remove anything stuck to injury (including clothing)
- DO NOT break blisters
- DO NOT remove loose skin
- DO NOT apply lotions, ointments, fatty substances, or use adhesive dressings on major burns
- ALWAYS apply cold water as above – to this can be added 4 drops per cupful of Hypercal Lotion as wash.

HOW TO USE: HERBS, PAGE 16 | HOMOEOPATHICS, PAGE 20 | CELL SALTS, PAGE 25

INTERNAL PROCEDURE FOR ALL BURNS

Homoeopathic

Arnica 30c: For shock, three times in one day. For major burns follow with Arnica 30c 4–5 times daily for a few days if necessary.

Cantharis 30c: For raw, smarting pain of burns and scalds. To calm and help relieve pain. Give every 10–15 minutes for the first hour, then as needed.

Causticum 30c: For painful burns that do not heal, that fester, or that break out after having healed.

EXTERNAL APPLICATIONS

Any of the following will soothe the burned surface of minor burns and complete the healing of major burns after critical period has passed: Calendula Cream, Urtica Urens Ointment or Tincture, Aloe Vera Gel, Vitamin E Oil squeezed from capsule, liquid Honey, Comfrey or Chickweed ointment or leaves.

Ointments can be applied directly to burn and covered with cloth or bandage. Tinctures (5 drops to $1/2$ cup of water) can be used to moisten cloth or bandage to cover the burned area lightly.

SEEK MEDICAL ADVICE

For all deep burns

For all burns covering more than 10 per cent of body surface

For burns to mouth or throat because swelling of the throat tissues can interfere with breathing

For large or numerous burns

For all burns around joints

For all burns from electrical currents

If pus forms on the burned surface

PREVENTION

Most burns can be prevented. Take special care.

- Do not let small babies go near a fire
- Keep matches, lamps and heaters out of reach

- Turn handles of pots on stove so children can't reach them
- Use short cords on electric jugs and have these in a holder so they can't be tipped over
- Use non-inflammable clothing
- Do not have hot tap on 'out' side of bath
- Always check water temperature before putting child in bath
- Play safe with the sun. Avoid excessive sunbathing – especially for fair-skinned children and at the beginning of the season. Use sunblock.

HOW TO USE: HERBS, PAGE 16 | HOMOEOPATHICS, PAGE 20 | CELL SALTS, PAGE 25

Chicken Pox

An infectious disease.

Transferred by droplets from mouth or nose. Shingles (Herpes Zoster) is often a source of contact. Usually a mild disease with characteristic skin eruptions; occasionally a child is very ill with it.

DESCRIPTION

Begins as itchy, red spots like flea bites, usually on the trunk. The spots enlarge, fill with fluid and turn to blisters. These eventually burst and develop into itchy scabs.

There is some discomfort and fever, loss of appetite and irritability. Common age for disease is under ten years, common season is autumn and winter.

Incubation period: about 15–20 days.

Isolation period: one week from the first sign of rash.

Recovery time: about two weeks.

WHAT TO DO

Keep the skin clean with frequent baths or showers, using Pine Oil soap or 2 tbsp of Baking Soda in the bath. Mix 3 drops of Lavender Oil with 2 tsp of Olive or Soya Oil and rub on affected skin.

Herbs

Good herbs for itch: Burdock and Sarsaparilla. Soak a cloth in an infusion made from these herbs, or add it to the bath water.

To calm itch: Yarrow, Chamomile and/or Lavender can be added to above herbs. They can also be drunk together as a tea.

Homoeopathic

After suspected contact: Rhus Tox 30c may help the child's resistance to the disease when given night and morning for three days (starting within two days of contact) then one dose per week for two weeks.

Antim Tart 30c: For early stages, spots slow in appearing, with bronchitis, sweats easily, is drowsy and peevish but wants company.

Pulsatilla 30c: Weepy child who is not thirsty despite fever.

Rhus Tox 30c: Itching is extreme, mental and physical restlessness.

Varicella 30c (Nosode, see page 31): To help clear a severe case or for lingering after-effects of the disease. *Do not give while disease is incubating.*

Cell Salts

Ferr Phos: When fever, irritability and discomfort are present.

Kali Mur: Alternate with Ferr Phos when fever stage is passing.

One dose of each every two hours for the first few days.

Calc Sulph: Where eruptions have yellow infected-looking discharge.

TO BUILD RESISTANCE

To strengthen the immune system and help restore to full health after the disease or vaccination see Resistance and Immunity, page 29.

HOW TO USE: HERBS, PAGE 16 | HOMOEOPATHICS, PAGE 20 | CELL SALTS, PAGE 25

Choking

Child's airways are partially or totally blocked by an obstruction, making breathing difficult or impossible. May occur when something goes down windpipe rather than food passage; when food is inadequately chewed and quickly swallowed; or when child has put something in his/her mouth and accidentally swallowed it.

DESCRIPTION

Difficulty in breathing; child will be unable to speak and may be gripping the throat; lips and mouth become blue; veins of face and neck become prominent.

WHAT TO DO

1. Remove any obvious obstruction to airways if possible.
2. *Baby:* Hold upside-down by the legs and give 3–4 smart knocks between shoulder blades using the heel of your hand. Take care *not* to hit too *hard*.

   If still choking, keeping head lower than body, place two fingers on centre of chest between the nipples and press down 1–1.25 cm (up to 0.5 inch) about 4 times.

   Repeat if necessary.

   If this does not dislodge the obstruction, see 4. below for older child. Be careful not to use too much pressure.
3. *Toddler:* Put child head-down across your arm or knee and, using the heel of your hand, give 4 knocks to the back between the shoulder blades.

   If still choking, turn child over, keeping head lower than body, place the heel of one hand on centre of the chest just below the nipples and press down 1.25–2cm (0.5–0.75 inches) 4 times.

   Repeat if necessary.

   If this does not dislodge the obstruction, see 4. below. Be careful not to use too much pressure.
4. *Older child:* Hug child from behind, using a clenched fist, applying sharp pressure just below front ribs to force the air upward and the object out.

Herbs

Scratched throat: Gargle with strong Sage tea.

SEEK FURTHER ADVICE

If vomiting or pains in the stomach develop;
if child is wheezing;
if object cannot be dislodged.

HOW TO USE: HERBS, PAGE 16 | HOMOEOPATHICS, PAGE 20 | CELL SALTS, PAGE 25

Cold

A cold is an inflammation of the mucous membranes of the nose and sinus passages caused by a number of viruses. While infections, dampness, draughts or changes of temperature do not cause a cold, they do weaken resistance to the cold viruses which children come in contact with so easily.

DESCRIPTION

Watery, nasal discharge, blocked nose, sneezing, sore throat, watery eyes and slight cough. Young children may have a fever as the body tries to throw off the virus. A simple cold usually subsides after a few days. (See also Fever, page 104)

WHAT TO DO

- Protect child from changes of temperature, dampness and draughts but do not overdress your child as this can aggravate the congestion.
- Have child soak in a warm bath to which is added 2 tbsp of Epsom Salts or powdered Ginger to open the pores and help release toxins from the bloodstream.

Herbs
The following can be used as a drink, a gargle, and/or added to bath water:

Antiseptic: Thyme and Sage

To soothe inflamed area: Coltsfoot

To open the pores and help reduce fever: Lemon Balm

To provide extra nourishment during the cold: Marjoram, Teatree, Thyme and/or Lavender can also be taken, mixed with honey if desired. (Honey can help healing if *not* heated above 45°C/113°F.)

To help build resistance: Regular herbal teas during the winter months also help to ward off the offending viruses. Take Vitamin A and C-rich herbs such as: Mullein, Parsley, Burdock, Rosehip, Comfrey, Yarrow and Liquorice.

Homoeopathic

As Homoeopathy deals with specific symptoms, please check under the relevant heading (e.g. Cough, Nose – Congestion, Throat (Sore)). For recurrent colds, or to help prevent a cold during the winter months, see Resistance and Immunity, page 29.

Cell Salts

Ferr Phos: Fever, dry nose, shivering, child can't get warm.
Calc Phos: Chronic tendency to take cold.
Calc Sulph: If sore throat is first sign of cold.
Kali Mur: If cold develops fully, with blocked nose, white tongue, greyish-white mucous or clear jelly-like mucous.
Kali Sulph: Fever with greenish-yellow nasal discharge.
Nat Mur: Watery, nasal discharge, sneezing.

SEE ALSO

Bronchitis, Asthma or Pneumonia: If noisy breathing or shortness of breath occur.
Cough: If cough becomes worse.
Measles: For runny nose when accompanied by sore throat and red, watery eyes.
Nose: If discharge becomes thick and yellow (may indicate an infection).
Throat and Mumps: If neck glands become swollen or sore.

HOW TO USE: HERBS, PAGE 16 | HOMOEOPATHICS, PAGE 20 | CELL SALTS, PAGE 25

Cold Sores

A virus (Herpes Simplex) which causes clusters of small fluid-like blisters to appear, usually on the lips or nostrils. It is often preceded by a burning sensation. The virus can be activated by sunlight, or by an upper respiratory tract infection. Also there may be a fever.

The sores dry to a scab in 5–10 days.

WHAT TO DO

- Dab Hypercal Lotion, Teatree Oil, Golden Seal Tincture, or Lemon Oil directly onto affected area frequently during the day
- Use diluted Golden Seal Tincture to rinse the mouth
- Apply ice to affected part to help relieve burning sensation.

Herbs
Deficiencies in Calcium and Vitamin D often accompany cold sores so use Chickweed, Dandelion, Puha, Rosehip and/or Parsley teas daily, especially if the cold sores often recur.

Homoeopathic
Arsen Alb 30c: Burning, itching and swelling of the sores. Also use for chronic tendency to cold sores.

Cantharis 30c: For large blisters which smart and burn.

Herpes Simplex nosode 30c: A dose taken at the end of an attack can help prevent recurrence.

Nat Mur 30c: Fever blisters, eruptions around mouth, may be on tongue and under nose.

Rhus Tox 30c: Corners of mouth ulcerate; blisters are angry-looking with great itching and tingling.

Cell Salts
Calc Fluor: Cold sores at corners of mouth.

Nat Mur: Blisters around mouth, cold sores on lip.

Conjunctivitis

The tissue that lines the eyelids and runs out over the eyeball is called the conjunctiva. Inflammation of this tissue, due to cold, irritation or germ, is called conjunctivitis.

DESCRIPTION

Burning and smarting of the eyelid. When eyelid is pulled away from eye lightly, the normally pink lid appears reddened. Tears may flood out although the child is not crying and there is often sensitivity to light. There may be a yellow discharge, especially evident upon waking with gummed eyes.

WHAT TO DO

Make a solution of Hypercal and/or Euphrasia Tincture (5 drops to $1/2$ glass of water). Moisten cotton wool balls with solution and use to rub away discharge. Sweep from inner to outer edge of the eye and be sure to use a new cotton ball for each sweep. When eye is clear, place 2 drops of same solution into infected eye. Place the drops carefully into inner corner of eye. Repeat eye-drops 3 times daily for 3–4 days.

Herbs
Use a weak solution of these herbs to bathe the eyes: Eyebright, Chamomile and/or Golden Seal. The same mixture can be taken as a tea.

Homoeopathic
Arsen Alb 30c: Intense sensitivity to light with heat and burning in eyes.
Belladonna 30c: Sudden, violent symptoms; swollen, staring, brilliant dilated eyes which are worse from exposure to heat and daylight. Eyes red, feel full of sand, better from rubbing.

HOW TO USE: HERBS, PAGE 16 | HOMOEOPATHICS, PAGE 20 | CELL SALTS, PAGE 25

Euphrasia 30c: Lids stuck together after sleep, constant thick, painful discharge with inclination to blink. Eyelids red and swollen. Tears scald and irritate cheeks.

Mercurius 30c: Profuse discharge which burns the cheeks; extreme intolerance of light.

Pulsatilla 30c: Yellow bland discharge; itchy, sore lids.

Cell Salts

Ferr Phos: First stage of inflammation.

Kali Sulph: Yellow-green coloured crusts on lids.

Nat Phos: Discharge of yellow mater; eyelids stuck together in morning.

Constipation

Retarded bowel action, causing either total absence or difficulty in the passage of faeces (stools).

Poor bowel habits begin in childhood. If the bowels do not move regularly (daily), the kidney, skin, liver, lungs and lymph have to work harder and eventually other health problems are created.

WHAT TO DO

Commercial laxatives can irritate the bowel, force peristaltic action, and tire the bowel muscle.

Drink adequate fluids: As a rule, find child's weight in kilograms, and give this amount of fluid ounces daily. To each glass of water can be added 1 drop of Rosemary Oil

Exercise regularly.

Increase dietary fibre with wholegrain breads and muesli.

Fresh Vegetables: Fresh beans, beetroot (top included), carrots, celery, lettuce and cucumber.

Fruits: Figs, prunes, pears, peaches, grapes, berries, pineapple.

Eliminate junk foods, white flour and sugar products and cheese.

On rising drink a glass of water which has the juice from $1/2$ lemon added to it.

- Cold-pressed Olive Oil (1 tsp–1 tbspn) should be included in the daily diet.
- Make homemade jelly using agar instead of gelatine (28 ml / 2 tbsp Agar to $1/2$ litre/17 fl oz of boiling water; half boiling water, half fruit juice; or rosehip tea). Flavour with honey or lemon juice. Served with fruit, this is easily taken by a child and helps to loosen the bowel motions. Can be taken daily.

Herbs

Liquorice, Rosemary, Linseed, Oatstraw, Borage and Senna. (When using Senna, always add a pinch of Ginger to alleviate the griping pains that Senna can cause. Do not use Senna for babies.)

HOW TO USE: HERBS, PAGE 16 | HOMOEOPATHICS, PAGE 20 | CELL SALTS, PAGE 25

Homoeopathic

Apis 30c: Shooting upward pains in rectum before or during bowel motion; often passes stool whilst urinating.

Bryonia 30c: Stools are dry, hard, large and difficult to pass.

Causticum 30c: Unsuccessful desire with pain and great straining. Easier to pass stool by standing.

Nat Mur 30c: Dry, crumbling stool, difficult to expel with bleeding and pain in rectum.

Nux Vomica 30c: Frequent, ineffectual urging, worse after party or overeating.

Psorinum 30c: For stubborn cases that do not respond to above remedies.

Cell Salts

Calc Fluor: Weak rectal muscles. Huge accumulation with anal cracks, very painful piles, great difficulty in expelling waste matter.

Ferr Phos: Constipation with inflammation, heat or pain and piles.

Kali Sulph: Constipation with yellow, slimy tongue.

Nat Mur: Constipation with headache, maybe haemorrhoids or sore feeling in anus after passing stool; dry stools difficult to pass.

Nat Phos: Alternates with diarrhoea, all efforts result in nothing.

Nat Sulph: Hard, knotty stools.

Silica: For pale children, bowel motion never seems completed.

Cough

Reflex expulsive action to remove foreign bodies or mucous from the breathing passages.

WHAT TO DO

For foreign objects see Choking (page 73).

Coughs usually go with a cold but can also herald more serious illness.

Herbs

Soothe the breathing passages with Marshmallow, Liquorice or Coltsfoot.

Strengthen the lungs against invading germs with Mullein, Hyssop, Comfrey or Teatree.

The cough may become looser at first, this is a sign of mucous loosening and being expelled. It should be encouraged, not suppressed.

Homoeopathic

The cough remedies are very specific to the individual case. We mention here only those remedies cited in our Health Kit. Further remedies can be found in the recommended homoeopathic books.

Aconite 30c: Worse for exposure to dry, cold weather; also worse from entering a warm room; short of breath, short, dry barking cough which wakes child from sleep. Little or no expectoration.

Antim Tart 30c: Whistling or rattling mucous with little expectoration; maybe pain in chest, drowsy and sweaty; must sit up to cough.

Arsen Alb 30c: Frequent sneezing, chilly, dry hacking cough with no expectoration; better if head is kept warm. Worse after midnight.

Bacillinum 30c: Lingering, stubborn or recurring coughs worse at night and early morning; recurring after antibiotics.

HOW TO USE: HERBS, PAGE 16 | HOMOEOPATHICS, PAGE 20 | CELL SALTS, PAGE 25

Belladonna 30c: Moaning and crying; burning, throbbing; tickling cough with blood-streaked mucous.

Bryonia 30c: Hard, hollow, very painful cough with raw throat and hoarse voice. Worse from eating and from warm room. Must hold chest during cough.

Gelsemium 30c: Summer colds and influenza-related coughs; sneezing and fullness at root of nose with headache, heavy eyes, maybe general aches.

Hepar Sulph 30c: Bouts of dry, hoarse suffocative coughs. Child is sensitive to touch, pain, draughts and cold, dry air. Almost chokes on the phlegm.

Lycopodium 30c: Deep, hollow, tickling cough. Worse 4–8 pm.

Nux Vomica 30c: Painful, spasmodic cough. Gagging and retching with bursting headache. Feels cold and likes to be covered.

Phosphorus 30c: Persistent cough affecting the throat; worse from talking and going from warm to cold air.

Pulsatilla 30c: Persistent cough that is dry in the evening and loose in the morning; better in the open air, some thick, frothy mucous.

Cell Salts

Calc Phos: Suffocating cough, better lying down. Any mucous is like raw egg white.

Ferr Phos: Will often cut short an attack which begins with a short, dry, tickling cough with no expectoration.

Kali Mur: Hoarse, croupy-sounding cough with white tongue and mucous.

Kali Sulph: Rattly cough with yellow, shiny mucous, worse in a warm room and evening; better in cool, open air.

Mag Phos: Cough sounds like whooping cough but with no discharge of mucous.

Nat Mur: Clear, watery, salty discharge which may come from eyes, nose or mouth, always accompanies cough.

Nat Sulph: Thick yellow-green mucous, worse in damp weather; pain in chest on coughing.

Silica: Thick, yellow-green mucous, worse from cold drinks and in the morning.

TYPES OF COUGH

Coughs can also indicate a more serious complaint; it is well to check the symptoms below and, where necessary, refer to the relevant page.

Asthma: Wheeze from deep in lungs, difficulty in expelling air, pounding in chest.

Bronchitis: May start as a cold but moves to the chest with rattly cough, feeling of tightness, maybe a slight temperature rise, yellow mucous may be coughed up.

Cold: Cough not severe, no shortness of breath or noisy breathing.

Croup: Loud, barking cough, noisy on breathing in, hoarse voice, shortness of breath.

Measles: The measles cough usually comes when other measles symptoms have developed.

Pneumonia: Very ill; rapid breathing, high temperature accompany cough.

Whooping Cough: Spasms of coughs in rapid succession; child cannot draw breath until spasm is over; this desperate sucking in of air causes the characteristic 'whoop'.

SEEK MEDICAL ADVICE

If the cough is getting worse, if your child can't swallow saliva, has any shortness of breath or problems with breathing.

HOW TO USE: HERBS, PAGE 16 | HOMOEOPATHICS, PAGE 20 | CELL SALTS, PAGE 25

Cramp

Violent muscle spasm in one or more muscles brought on by interference with circulation to the part.

Cramp can be caused by one of the following: overuse; excessive jarring or tearing of muscles; poor circulation, resulting in inability to deliver essential nutrients (especially Calcium, Magnesium and Vitamins) to the body. This is especially common during pregnancy.

DESCRIPTION

Muscle knots and shortens, causing sharp, grabbing pain and stiffness. Muscle cannot be used during spasm. Cramps are often worse in the afternoon, in hot weather or during sleep.

WHAT TO DO

- Gentle stretching
- Light feather touch to affected part
- Alternate hot and cold packs (hot-water bottle or hot flannel and ice-filled flannel) always ending with a cold pack.

For recurring cramps: Avoid low-calcium foods like meat, liver, wheat and citrus (which robs the body of calcium); eat more millet, sesame seed, yoghurt, oats, milk, alfalfa sprouts.

If cramps are a result of salt loss, replace by drinking flat lemonade or electrolyte solution as a temporary measure (500 ml/17 fl oz boiled water, 8 tsp sugar, $1/2$ tsp salt). However, it is more important to correct the mineral imbalance (see below).

Herbs

Recurrent problems indicate a mineral imbalance, so drink herbs rich in Calcium, Magnesium and Vitamins C and E: Valerian, Dandelion, Comfrey, Thyme, Chamomile, Yellow Dock and Sage.

Stomach Cramps: Use one or more of the following: Peppermint, Chamomile, Fennel Seed, Catnip and/or ground Cloves. Apply a few drops of Teatree Oil externally to the affected area.

Homoeopathic

Calc Carb 30c: Helps to remove a tendency to cramps.

Cocculus 30c: Cramps in chest.

Colocynth 30c: Cramp in hip or stomach, causing child to bend double.

Cuprum 30c: For cramps in calves, soles and palms.

Lycopodium 30c: Cramps in toes, calves and fingers.

Cell Salts

Calc Phos: If cramps occur during teething.

Mag Phos: Main remedy for sudden cramps.

HOW TO USE: HERBS, PAGE 16 | HOMOEOPATHICS, PAGE 20 | CELL SALTS, PAGE 25

Croup

Juvenile form of laryngitis, usually caused by a virus creating an infection in the larynx region.

DESCRIPTION

Starts as a mild upper respiratory infection, with some hoarseness. Then child wakes at night, clutches at throat with difficult breathing, husky voice and characteristic dry, barking cough. This lasts half an hour to three hours and then suddenly eases. Croup is very rare under six months and usually occurs between the ages of two and four.

WHAT TO DO

Croup without a fever: Treat by filling the room with steam (boil kettle or run hot tap in bathroom). Reassure and stay with child. A few drops of Teatree, Eucalyptus and/or Lavender Oil may be added to steaming water. Check breathing 2–3 hours after attack. Keep the room warm for the next few nights.

Croup with a fever: This is more serious as it is accompanied by a chest cold. Breathing difficulty comes on more slowly but can come any time; steaming only partly relieves.

Herbs

Give frequent sips of hot Lemon/Mint drinks sweetened with honey if necessary; give child a bath to which has been added 2 tsp Ginger powder or 2 tsp baking soda.

Sip frequently a warm herb drink made from any or all of the following: Lemon, Thyme, Mullein, Catnip and/or Garlic. Add one drop of Lobelia Tincture for each year of the child's life (some children react strongly if larger amounts are given). These herbs help to soothe and calm the breathing passages and help fight any infection.

Homoeopathic

A common approach is to alternate Aconite, Hepar Sulph and Spongia at 15-minute intervals until relief is obtained.

Aconite 30c: Child is restless and anxious; after exposure to cold dry winds, cough becomes hard, dry and barking.

Hepar Sulph 30c: Chilly and sweaty; loose rattling cough; worse from least uncovering.

Spongia 30c: Noisy, rasping tight cough without wheeze or rattle; maybe tough phlegm difficult to cough up and usually swallowed; breathing is harsh.

Note: If throat is swollen so that child is choking and lips have a blue tinge seek medical help.

Cell Salts

Alternate Ferr Phos and Kali Mur. Add the following if necessary.

Calc Sulph: If croup is recurrent. Take regularly for several weeks.

Mag Phos: Great difficulty in breathing.

SEEK MEDICAL ADVICE

If, when child breathes in, the abdominal wall draws in more than a little. This means there is considerable lung obstruction.

If noisy breathing persists and child is unable to swallow, or if child becomes blue, restless and struggles very hard to breathe. (This child would need hospitalization.)

HOW TO USE: HERBS, PAGE 16 | HOMOEOPATHICS, PAGE 20 | CELL SALTS, PAGE 25

Diarrhoea

Occurs when the normal rate of movement of waste matter through the digestive tract is sped up or if absorption in the bowels is inhibited by disease; the contents will still be liquid when they reach the rectum and so loose motions result.

Acute diarrhoea can be caused by: infections either in the gut or outside the gut (i.e. tonsillitis, ear infections, urinary infections); anxiety or fear; irritants taken into the stomach and bowel via food; laxatives; metabolic disturbance, e.g. nutritional deficiency, allergic reactions, weakened digestive organs; antibiotic treatment; unripe, greasy foods. The poorly nourished child is the most prone to diarrhoea.

Diarrhoea that goes on for more than a few days must always be investigated by a medical doctor.

WHAT TO DO

1. Take no foods for twenty-four hours.
2. Alternate hot and cold compresses to abdomen if painful (use hot flannel or hot-water bottle, and ice wrapped in flannel).
3. Take plenty of fluids. *It is important to guard against dehydration caused by excessive fluid-loss through the bowel.* Any or all of the following can be taken throughout the day:

   Water with Oil of Clove or Rosemary (1 drop only of each to a cup of water)

   Chamomile Tea

   Cold Black Tea

   Electrolyte Solution (500 ml/17 fl oz boiled water, 8 tsp sugar, $^1/_2$ tsp salt)

   Kaolin-Pectin mixture: Stocked by chemists. Prevents absorption of bacterial toxins by forming a film on the intestinal wall. Also absorbs some of the toxins. The nutrients are quickly firmed up and temporary relief is provided. However, it is still wise to provide nutritional fluids wherever possible. When camping or away from home, cool flat (by heating) lemonade is useful and readily available.

If breastfeeding, continue and add fluid drinks as directed for mother and/or baby.

4. Sustaining drinks:

Vegetable drink: Cut 2–5 vegetables into small pieces and bring to the boil in enough water to leave 2–3 cupfuls of juice. Simmer for 20–30 minutes. This can be taken warm or cold throughout the day and supplies adequate vitamins and minerals. Best vegetables are potato (just thickly peeled skins), parsnip, sweet potato, parsley.

Fruit drink: Blend organic apples in blender for apple sauce, or cut up apples (pips and skins included) and boil in enough water to leave 2–3 cups of juice. Pulp can be kept as a first solid after 24-hour fast is complete.

Grain drink: Simmer 60 gm (2^1/$_2$ oz) barley, rice or oatmeal in 500 ml (17 fl oz) of water for 30 minutes, then strain.

5. *First foods:* If your child is distressingly hungry and dissatisfied with fluids, give grated raw apple including pips (no other raw fruit should be taken) for the older child every two hours. For the younger child, make a Slippery Elm porridge and mix with any or all of the following: stewed apple, bananas, ginger, carob, cinnamon or nutmeg (until bowels firm up).

Dry crackers or rice may also be useful for the older child.

Herbs

For stomach pains: Calendula, Catnip, Fennel Seed, Peppermint or Slippery Elm.

To help tonify the system: Gentian or Rhubarb Root, Comfrey.

As antiseptic against bacteria: Golden Seal.

Take with meals: 1 drop of Clove or Rosemary Essential Oil in water.

Homoeopathic

Arsen Alb 30c: Diarrhoea may be caused by spoiled foods or too much fruit. Frequent scanty, offensive stools which burn the skin. Great exhaustion follows stools.

Calc Phos 30c: Green, slimy, undigested stools, worse during teething. Noisy, spluttering stools.

China 30c: Debilitating, involuntary, painless, diarrhoea with putrid smell. Worse after eating fruit.

HOW TO USE: HERBS, PAGE 16 | HOMOEOPATHICS, PAGE 20 | CELL SALTS, PAGE 25

Colocynth 30c: Diarrhoea with colic, better from bending double. Worse from slightest food or drink.

Gelsemium 30c: Diarrhoea yellow and changeable, brought on by nerves, fright or excitement.

Hepar Sulph 30c: Clay-coloured, sour-smelling stools.

Mercurius 30c: Slimy, bloody stools. Never-get-done feeling.

Podophyllum 30c: Morning stool, painless watery yellow and profuse and gushing. Worse after eating and drinking. Maybe a natural stool later in day.

Rhus Tox 30c: If recurring problem. May have no appetite. May be worse from apple juice.

Veratrun Alb 30c: Watery painful diarrhoea with stomach cramps and chilly.

Cell Salts

Calc Phos: If diarrhoea occurs during teething.

Ferr Phos: Undigested stools come on suddenly with fever.

Kali Mur: Pale-coloured stools, worse from rich foods.

Kali Phos: Foul-smelling diarrhoea.

Kali Sulph: Yellow stools and cramps.

LONG-TERM APPROACH

Cut down on white flour products, meat, salt and pepper.

Be sure to include plenty of live natural yoghurt to replace friendly bacteria to the intestines.

Check the cleanliness of the household.

Protect food from flies.

Wash hands.

Wash baby bottles, etc, thoroughly.

See medical practitioner for intestinal parasites. There are homoeopathic Nosodes to act against these. Seek homoeopathic advice.

SEEK MEDICAL AID

If child shows signs of dehydration; i.e. skin does not rebound on pinching lightly.

If child appears limp, pale and unaware of surroundings.

---

1 Glue Ear

An accumulation of thick mucous in the middle ear. Hearing is lessened, child often talks more loudly than usual. There is usually no pain.

Glue ear of itself is not necessarily a problem but it can make ear infections more likely. Time may eventually clear the narrow passages, but any hearing loss must be carefully checked and treated.

WHAT TO DO

Herbs

To help break down mucous in any part of the body: Comfrey, Bayberry, Queens Delight, Fenugreek, Golden Seal, Elecampane and Coltsfoot.

Homoeopathic

Calc Carb 30c: Difficult hearing with cracking noises in ear and full feeling.

Kali Mur 30c: For catarrhal conditions of the middle ear where child hears cracking noises and ear feels congested on swallowing or blowing nose.

Kali Sulph 30c: Deafness with discharge of yellow matter.

Merc Dulcis 30c: Blocked Eustachian tube, offensive breath; difficult hearing, worse during a cold.

Pulsatilla 30c: Difficult hearing as if ear were stuffed. Maybe some thick, bland discharge.

Other remedies are best chosen by a competent homoeopath, so seek advice if none of the above remedies are suitable.

See Remedy Pictures – Homoeopathic (page 199).

HOW TO USE: HERBS, PAGE 16 | HOMOEOPATHICS, PAGE 20 | CELL SALTS, PAGE 25

Cell Salts

Alternate Ferr Phos and Kali Mur for deafness following a cold.
Calc Sulph: For difficult hearing with thick, yellow discharge.

2 Hearing

- If a child does not respond to quiet, unexpected noises by six months, if there is little babbling by one year, or if there is any doubt in your mind about your child's hearing ability, a proper hearing test is appropriate. These are available through your GP or health visitor.

    A competent homoeopath may be able to provide some assistance with this problem. Success with homoeopathic remedies largely depends on the cause of the hearing difficulty.

- On the inside of the eardrum, the middle ear must stay full of air to transmit sounds efficiently from the eardrum to the hearing nerve. When fluid fills this space, caused by a blockage in the tube leading to the nose, tone and hearing are lessened. If this space is constantly fluid-filled, a 'glue-ear' develops, and if bacteria invade this area, an ear infection develops.

3 Middle Ear Infection

Child is sick, irritable, has earache and usually tugs on ear. Partial hearing loss. Red and angry-looking eardrum. Usually associated with a cold, as nasal blockage causes middle eardrum to fill with fluid. It can also accompany measles or bronchitis, or be caused through excessive swimming.

An ear infection that is left will either clear by a reopening of the nasal passages or by perforation of the eardrum, causing a gooey, yellow-white fluid to flow out of the ear. This perforation will almost always heal by itself but if it happens several times, there can be scarring on the eardrum which lessens hearing ability. It is therefore important that each infection be completely cleared to help prevent repeated infections and hearing damage.

Complications of an untreated ear infection can in some cases be mastoiditis or meningitis.

WHAT TO DO – Acute Ear Infection

Have your doctor monitor the state of the eardrum during the infection.

Herbs

To help ease the pain: Lobelia Tincture (1 drop for every year of child's age – 5 drops maximum). Some children react strongly to this herb, so it is wise to use a low dose. Give on a teaspoon with water internally at 15-minute intervals.

Further pain relief: May be obtained with 1 drop of Mullein Oil or Lemon Oil placed on a warm teaspoon with 10–20 drops of pure Olive Oil and poured into the ear duct. (Unless there are signs of perforated ear drum – intense pain or discharge from the ear.)

To help purify blood and cleanse the ear canal: Golden Seal and Queens Delight.

To calm and induce sleep: Elder and Chamomile.

Homoeopathic

Aconite 30c: For acute onset in an otherwise healthy child. Redness and pain better from hot applications. Very thirsty.

Belladonna 30c: Sudden and throbbing pain, with red, hot face worse from least jar or knock.

Chamomilla 30c: Child is angry, cross and wants to be carried. Worse from heat. Cannot tolerate pain. One cheek red, the other pale.

Hepar Sulph 30c: Hot, maybe itching ear with sore throat, pus discharge, worse in a draught, sensitive to touch.

Kali Bich 30c: Tearing pains or sharp stitches in ears following congestion in nose and throat.

Mercurius 30c: Discharge can be thick or thin, but always streaked with blood; boils in external canal, worse from warmth of bed.

Merc Dulcis 30c: Blocked Eustachian tube, infection with offensive breath and difficult hearing.

Pulsatilla 30c: Ear feels stuffed, sharp pulsating pains, discharge is thick and bland, better in the open air, worse in a warm room, and at night.

See also Remedy Pictures – Homoeopathic (page 199).

HOW TO USE: HERBS, PAGE 16 | HOMOEOPATHICS, PAGE 20 | CELL SALTS, PAGE 25

Cell Salts

Calc Phos: Earache with swelling of glands about the ear and maybe a clear discharge.

Ferr Phos: For throbbing, burning pain; external ear may be red and hot.

Kali Mur: Swollen glands and Eustachian tubes; noises in ears on blowing nose.

Kali Sulph: Earache with thin, yellow discharge, yellow coating on tongue and sharp pains.

Mag Phos: Earache with sharp, shooting pains.

See also Remedy Pictures – Cell Salts (page 210).

WHAT TO DO – Long-term Treatment

If infections are not completely cleared they will recur.

Check for food allergy, especially dairy products (see Allergy).

For incomplete return to health after infectious diseases such as mumps, see page 29 (Resistance).

Herbs

Drink herbs daily to detoxify the ear canal: Queens Delight, Elecampane or Burdock.

As an antiseptic: Golden Seal.

To help loosen and move the mucous: Comfrey or Fenugreek.

These herbs will need to be continued for at least three weeks.

Homoeopathic

Calc Carb 30c: Chronic enlarged glands, pressing, throbbing, cracking noises, worse from slightest cold about neck and ears.

Causticum 30c: Wax, middle ear catarrh, blocked feeling. Roaring rushing noises or re-echoing of sounds in ears.

Medorrhinum 30c: Pains and deafness associated with chronic catarrhal conditions in children.

Parotidinum 30c: If ear problems have lingered since child had mumps.

Streptococcin 30c: Constantly recurring infections with history of streptococcal infection.

You should see a homoeopath for advice.

Cell Salts

As for *Acute Infections*.

Also Calc Sulph: If there is a thick, yellow or bloody discharge.

4 Outer Ear Infection

Infection of the skin lining, eardrum or outer ear canal. Causes pain, itching and discharge from the ear, often with reduced hearing because the ear canal is blocked.

WHAT TO DO

Don't ever use cotton-wool buds to penetrate the ear canal as the wax lining will protect the skin surface and absorb germs and bacteria, thereby preventing fungal growth. The blockage will clear itself during the healing process.

Homoeopathic

Belladonna 30c: Red, swollen and painful to touch.

Calc Carb 30c: Eruption on and behind ear; enlarged glands.

Causticum 30c: Helps to break down accumulated wax.

Graphites 30c: Moisture and eruption behind ears.

Hepar Sulph 30c: Itching in ears, pus discharge.

Mezereum 30c: Ears feel much too open as of a cold wind; likes to bore fingers into ears.

Pulsatilla 30c: External ear is swollen and red.

See also Remedy Pictures – Homoeopathic (page 199).

5 Object in Ear

If ear drum is NOT perforated, flood ear with tepid water (symptoms of perforation: intense pain and discharge and possible decrease in hearing); have child tip head so that water flows upwards, not towards the drum. If this does not dislodge the object, seek further advice.

HOW TO USE: HERBS, PAGE 16 | HOMOEOPATHICS, PAGE 20 | CELL SALTS, PAGE 25

Insects can often be floated out with warm olive oil (temperature: so that spoon feels comfortable against your own upper lip).

Give Aconite 30c if needed for agitation.
Give Arnica 30c two doses before and two doses after any surgical treatment.

6 Wax in Ears

Do not attempt to clear wax during an infection.

Using a teaspoon of warm Olive Oil (temperature: so the spoon feels comfortable against your own upper lip). Have child place his/her head on pillow with affected ear up, pull earlobe up and back and pour Olive Oil in gently until canal is full. Press firmly on mound in front of ear. Pumping action forces the oil in between the wax. Have child remain in this position for ten minutes, then allow oil to drain out. Only do this if there is no history of perforation.

Homoeopathic
Causticum 30c: To break down accumulation of ear wax.

Eczema

Starts as itchy, red skin; may weep clear fluid after it is scratched. This forms crusts when it dries. If untreated, the skin becomes less red, dry and thickened. Often it starts on cheeks or forehead in babies; bends of knees or elbows in toddlers. It is not contagious.

Causes can be any of the following:

- Sensitivity or allergy to something contacted or eaten.
- Faulty metabolism, constipation, poor elimination of toxins.
- Nutritional deficiencies.

WHAT TO DO

We advise that you seek the help of an experienced natural health practitioner. Natural remedies can offer significant help to eczema sufferers.

Determine irritating agent – see Allergy.

Treat emotional aspects with Bach Flowers – a stressful situation can be sufficient to trigger a recurrence of eczema. (Books on Bach Flower Remedies are available at most health shops.)

Good foods to eat: avocado, dandelion, melons, sunflower seeds and goat's milk.

Check for presence of Candida Albicans (see Thrush, page 175, for more information).

Externally

- Avoid washing with regular soaps and shampoos, or using baby oils. Bathe affected parts often with plain water. Afterwards rub with a slice of cucumber. Apply lanolin-based ointment fortified with Vitamin A and E oils or pure Aloe Vera Gel.
- Mix one part Sage Oil with ten parts Olive Oil and apply locally.
- Dusting with Whey Powder can be soothing.
- Sea water can be beneficial, especially combined with careful exposure to the sun.

HOW TO USE: HERBS, PAGE 16 | HOMOEOPATHICS, PAGE 20 | CELL SALTS, PAGE 25

- For a hot inflamed type of eczema, add $1/4$ cup baking soda to bath 2–3 times weekly and soak in it for 15 minutes.
- For a dry, itchy type of eczema, add $1/4$ cup powdered ginger to bath 2–3 times weekly and soak in it for 15 minutes.

Herbs

These may cause an initial worsening of the condition due to increased elimination of toxins. Do not introduce any new creams at the same time as it may interfere with the cleansing process.

Blood purifiers: Burdock, Dandelion, Yellow Dock, Elecampane, Echinacea and/or Sassafras.

Bowel cleaners: Black Walnut or Rosemary.

Homoeopathic

Arsen Alb 6c: Chronic dry eczema with great burning and itching, thickened skin.

Graphites 6c: Raw behind ears, hands, elbow and knee flexures; cracks in nipples, toes, mouth or anus. Sticky, scabby eruptions oozing a gluey, honey-like fluid.

Nat Mur 6c: Raw, red and inflamed. Worse or better from eating salt or at the seashore.

Psorinum 6c: Intolerable itching all night, inherited tendency. Erupts on bends of joints with itching. Worse from warmth of bed. Very greasy, dirty-looking skin.

Rhus Tox 6c: Acute intense itching and tingling; red, swollen, circular-shaped and scaly; better from warm applications.

Sulphur 6c: Dry and scaly; itching and burning; worse from scratching and washing, every injury becomes infected. Skin troubles may alternate with intestinal problems.

There may be an initial worsening of symptoms due to increased elimination of toxins. Discontinue remedy immediately if this occurs and wait for things to settle down.

Cell Salts

Kali Mur: Skin has white, dry scales.

Kali Phos: Good for nervous children; skin is raw and sore.

Kali Sulph. Discharge is yellow-looking.

Nat Mur: Watery eruptions worse in folds such as elbows and knees; skin is itchy, dry and cracked.

Eyes

1 Object in Eye

- If object is embedded in the eyeball, *do not* attempt to remove. Give Aconite 30c for shock and irritation and SEEK MEDICAL ADVICE.
- If object is freely moving in the eye, hold eyelids open, and using a cotton bud or corner of a clean handkerchief, gently wipe object from eye.
- If child will not allow this, place one drop of Castor Oil in eye to move object. After it is removed, apply firm pressure over closed eye using a soft pad such as a folded clean handkerchief.
- If eye is painful and child will not allow you to touch it, it is best to get your GP or local hospital to use pain-relieving eye drops and remove it for you.
- If bleeding from eye, bathe with Hypercal solution (made with five drops to $1/2$ glass of water, or one drop to an eyebath of water). Then seek medical help.
- If eye remains bloodshot or sore over the next few days, take Ruta Grav 30c three times during the day.

2 Blow to Eye

All blows to the eye are potentially serious
- If very severe, *do not examine* as this may aggravate the situation. Rest in lying down position. Apply cold compress immediately. Make compress (see page 19) using Comfrey or Eyebright; or Arnica Tincture (diluted five drops to $1/2$ cup of water).
- Keep eye covered with dressing but do not apply pressure.

HOW TO USE: HERBS, PAGE 16 | HOMOEOPATHICS, PAGE 20 | CELL SALTS, PAGE 25

Take Arnica 30c internally for a few days to reduce the blackening
and swelling.

3 Stye

An infection at the base of hairs that form eyelashes. Starts as redness and tender swelling, then pus forms and can discharge. Conjunctivitis can develop.

WHAT TO DO

At first feeling of tenderness or redness, gently pull at eyelashes.
This can remove the loose hair and irritation sometimes subsides.
Make a solution with 10 drops of Hypercal or Euphrasia Tincture in
$1/2$ a glass of water (or one drop to eyebath) and wash eye and eyelid
at least three times daily.

Herbs
Eye can be bathed with Chamomile tea.
Eyebright, Golden Seal and Bayberry can be taken together as a tea
3–4 times daily. These herbs are all beneficial for the eyes.

Homoeopathic
Aconite 30c: Inflamed from cold and feels like sand is in the eye.
    Worse from cold dry winds. Sensitive to light.
Apis 30c: To help prevent recurrence.
Graphites 30c: Red, swollen lids, worse from light.
Hepar Sulph 30c: For chronic stye problems. Worse from cold air
    and cold applications.
Pulsatilla 30c: For styes on the lower lid. Thick yellow bland dis-
    charge.
Silica 30c: Swollen tear ducts, worse from sunlight. Pustular condi-
    tion about eyes.
Sulphur 30c: Burning ulceration of lids.

Cell Salts
Silica.

4 Blocked Tear Duct

There are more tears in one eye and there may be yellow discharge.

WHAT TO DO

Gently massage down cheek from inner lower edge of eye below tear duct. Repeat twice daily.

Homoeopathic
Calc Carb 30c: Eye waters more in open air and early morning.
Nat Mur 30c: If discharge is more yellow and irritating.

Cell Salts
Nat Mur.

5 Eyestrain and Poor Vision

Some children complain of tired eyes after school or television. Some children with poor vision never complain – so ensure your child's vision is checked at school and learn to make your own observations. Watch for:

● Difficulty reading the blackboard
● Holding books very close to the eyes
● Sitting very close to the television
● Developing headaches or pain around eyes.

WHAT TO DO

Eye exercises and Touch for Health techniques can be useful. See an instructor.

HOW TO USE: HERBS, PAGE 16 | HOMOEOPATHICS, PAGE 20 | CELL SALTS, PAGE 25

Herbs

To relieve eyestrain: Eyebright, Golden Seal and Bayberry. (A weaker tea made from these can also be used as an eyewash.)

To strengthen: Jaborandi, Parsley or Chaparral. Vitamin A has a specific affinity for the eyes.

Homoeopathic

Should be treated by a homeopath *after* a sight test. It might indicate a wider problem.

Cell Salts

Calc Fluor: Blurred vision from eyestrain.
Ferr Phos: Pain from overstraining eyes.
Kali Phos: Weak eyesight from ill-health.

6 Squint

The eyes look in different directions at the same time.

Homoeopathic

Belladonna 30c: Squint sometimes with staring, fiery eyes in an excitable child.

Cicuta 30c: Spasmodic squint, pupils can move behind upper lids when head bends back.

7 Danger Signs with Eyes

SEEK PROFESSIONAL ADVICE

For any wound, cut or foreign body that enters eyeball.

For a painful greyish spot on cornea with redness around cornea.

For pain inside eye – iritis or glaucoma.

For difference in pupil size, especially with pain or headache.

For vision changing or fading.

For any inflammation or infection that fails to respond to treatment (whether medical or natural).

If condition fails to respond to above procedures.

Fever

When the body is upset by some invasion, whether the common cold virus or something more serious, the temperature will rise.

All healing processes speed up during a fever – the heart carrying blood, the respiration increasing oxygen uptake. Fever is not an enemy to be suppressed, but a signal that the body is working to ward off an invasion. With children under five years, a rise in temperature can produce a Febrile Convulsion (see Fits), so it is important to keep the temperature below danger level whilst not suppressing it entirely.

Mild Fever: 37.5–38.3°C (99.5–101°F)
Moderate Fever: 38.3–39.4°C (101–103°F)
High: 39.4°C (103°F). This temperature should be lowered quickly.
Extremely High: Over 40°C (104°F). This temperature must be cooled at once, to avoid convulsions.

Some children suffer fits at a temperature deemed mild.

WHAT TO DO

- Cool: Strip child to underclothes; if still hot to touch, sponge gently with *tepid* water or put in a tepid bath. Extreme cooling by cold baths causes the body to react against being chilled, i.e. triggers the heating mechanisms.
- Give child frequent, small drinks of water and herbal teas (see below).
- Find the cause of the fever and take steps to correct this.

Herbs
Herbs are best hot and frequent for fevers.

Laxative herbs to help eliminate toxic matter through the bowel: Senna, Thyme or Liquorice. Use these only if the child is constipated.

HOW TO USE: HERBS, PAGE 16 | HOMOEOPATHICS, PAGE 20 | CELL SALTS, PAGE 25

To help bring down fever: Yarrow, Lemon Balm, Catnip and/or Ginger.

To the bath: Add 1–2 tbsps Ginger powder or Epsom Salts; or 2–3 drops of Oils of Peppermint, Sage and/or Thyme.

Homoeopathic

Homoeopathic remedies provide a good first action that may often allay a more serious illness.

Aconite 30c: Sudden onset in a normally healthy child. Intensely nervous, restless, anxious. Skin is dry and hot with full, bounding pulse. Red cheeks; chilly on slightest movement. Great thirst.

Antim Tart 30c: Shivering with fever, pale face, thirst for little sips often. Chilly with short burst of heat.

Arsen Alb 30c: Patient is fearful and restless, burning pains relieved by warmth. Very thirsty for frequent sips, rapid prostration and increasing weakness.

Belladonna 30c: Sudden, violent onset. Flushed face, high temperature, pulse strong and rapid. Little or no thirst, may be delirious. Dry, burning hot skin, sparkling eyes.

Bryonia 30c: Fever with intense headache; prefers to lie still. Worse from least movement, even moving eyes. Very thirsty for large drinks of water. Pale and quiet. White coating down middle of tongue.

China 30c: May help the child who develops a fever easily and often.

Gelsemium 30c: Chilly, aches all over. Dizzy; does not want to move, dull headache, droopy eyes, heavy limbs, no thirst.

Mercurius 30c: Alternatively hot and cold. Profuse perspiration with no relief. Worse at night.

Rhus Tox 30c: Great weakness and prostration but extremely restless. Mental confusion, thickly-coated tongue, but red at tip, great thirst.

Cell Salts

Ferr Phos: First remedy for high temperature. Gradual onset. Red cheeks and throbbing head. Fast pulse. Better from cold applications to head.

Kali Phos: For those with a nervous temperature, this seems more effective than Ferr Phos.

SEEK MEDICAL ADVICE

If temperature remains elevated despite procedure or if you are worried.

See also Fits, page 107.

HOW TO USE: HERBS, PAGE 16 | HOMOEOPATHICS, PAGE 20 | CELL SALTS, PAGE 25

Fits

Fits or convulsions occur when the brain sends out jumbled messages to the muscles, making them move in uncontrolled ways. Fits usually last only a few minutes and are not uncommon between six months and three years, but are rare after five years. They are usually accompanied by a fever.

If children have had one fever fit, they are more susceptible to such fits. (If your child is having fits frequently without any sign of fever, then epilepsy is a possibility – seek medical, homoeopathic or naturopathic advice.)

Convulsions can occur during meningitis (see Meningitis).

DESCRIPTION

Child can sometimes be only slightly unwell and temperature rises very quickly. During the fit, the child goes stiff, eyes roll back, breathing is laboured, body twitches and shakes, child may turn blue around lips or bite tongue.

Child becomes unconscious, may vomit or soil himself; body relaxes and as he regains consciousness he is confused. After a sleep he wakens fully recovered.

WHAT TO DO

- Keep child *cool* (with fever fits this is most important – see Fever)
- Place gently on side (in recovery or coma position) to prevent choking
- Remove anything from in front of child's mouth
- Ensure he cannot hurt himself
- Remove tight clothing from neck
- After fit has finished, reassure and comfort child.

DURING FIT

Herbs

Place on tongue: 1–2 drops of Chamomile, Valerian, Lavender or Skullcap Tincture. Repeat every few minutes.

Homoeopathic

Aconite 30c: If convulsions are caused by a fright. Rigid and stiff with bright red face, foaming at mouth, crying out in sleep.

Belladonna 30c: Violent onset with large, glazed pupils.

Cuprum 30c: Violent convulsions with contraction of jaws; may begin in fingers or toes. Blue face and mouth. Gurgling in throat.

Ignatia 30c: For child who becomes hysterical due to grief, worry, jealousy, or after punishment. Twitching muscles.

Zincum 30c: Convulsion following infection or fever.

Cell Salts

Place on tongue one crushed Mag Phos tablet; follow in a few minutes with Calc Phos. Continue to alternate during convulsion and follow with 2–3 doses afterwards as well.

LONG-TERM APPROACH

If your child has had any fits, give daily drinks of Skullcap, Valerian and/or Passionflower to calm the nervous system. Continue thirty days.

SEEK MEDICAL ADVICE

If it is child's first fever fit.

If child comes out of one fit and goes straight into another, despite above procedure.

If child continues to fit despite above procedure.

HOW TO USE: HERBS, PAGE 16 | HOMOEOPATHICS, PAGE 20 | CELL SALTS, PAGE 25

Fractures

After a child has had a fall, check for the following:

- Painful swelling in any area other than bruised part
- One point of extreme tenderness over a bone
- A change in body shape on one side but not the other
- Child is unable to use a limb
- If pulse cannot be felt beyond an injury.

WHAT TO DO

1. If child has severe bleeding or shows signs of shock always deal with these first (see Wounds).
2. SEEK MEDICAL HELP URGENTLY.
3. Immobilize injured part by strapping firmly with strips of cloth or nappies and supporting limb wherever possible with splint e.g. rolled up newspaper), or strap to uninjured part of body.
4. Support in an elevated position when possible.
5. Never put an exposed broken bone (compound fracture) back into the wound – expert aid is required to thoroughly clean the area.

Herbs

Internally to help broken bones heal:
To calm nerves and ease pain: Chamomile or Valerian.
To help heal: Comfrey.
To ensure adequate Calcium and Magnesium during healing: Basil and Parsley.

External application:
To help swelling, deformity and unnatural mobility: Apply Comfrey Ointment to unbroken skin.

Homoeopathic

Arnica 30c: 3–4 times daily for first three days.
Symphytum 6x: Take twice daily for the first three weeks to help unite fracture.

Cell Salts

Calc Phos: To help unite fracture.

Alternate with Ferr Phos when there is redness and/or swelling around injury.

HOW TO USE: HERBS, PAGE 16 | HOMOEOPATHICS, PAGE 20 | CELL SALTS, PAGE 25

Headache

Headache can be caused by any of the following: spinal problems, visual strain, blood sugar problems, stress, muscular tension, digestive disturbances, allergies, sinusitis, dehydration or infection, e.g. influenza, measles.

A *migraine* is a severe headache often occurring at regular intervals, often one-sided and accompanied by nausea, vomiting and maybe preceded or accompanied by visual disturbances.

WHAT TO DO

The information here applies to both headaches and migraines. If you suspect a spinal or neck problem, check with a qualified osteopath or chiropractor.

Dietary changes may be necessary but such changes vary from person to person. See Allergy, or seek advice from a naturopath, homoeopath or Touch for Health instructor. Simple avoidance of fried foods, sugar products and dairy products may help, and remember to drink small amounts of water often.

Herbs
Choose at least one from each of the following categories and make a tea to be sipped often during headache.

For nerves: Valerian, Skullcap, Passionflower or Thyme.
To regulate blood sugar and liver action: Meadowsweet, Dandelion, Mandrake and/or Golden Seal.
To strengthen and harmonize the digestive system: Fennel, Sage, Rosemary, Thyme, Lavender and/or Peppermint.
Externally to soothe: A few drops of Oil of Rose or Lemongrass in the bath.

Homoeopathic
Argentum Nit 30c: Head feels extremely large; dizziness, better for pressure to head.
Belladonna 30c: Hot head; throbbing flushed face and cold feet; right front of head worse for lying down, uncovering, light,

noise, jar; better for holding head still or bending head backwards.

Bryonia 30c: Bursting, splitting frontal ache; extends backwards down neck and shoulders. Worse for moving eyes, and in the morning.

China 30c: Head feels as if brain is bouncing within skull. Better from bending double.

Gelsemium 30c: Heavy eyelids, dull heavy ache with dizziness; tight band feeling around head, worse from emotion or bad news.

Nat Mur 30c: Blinding headache with pale face and nausea, preceded by numbness and tingling in lips, tongue and nose. Worse from eyestrain, better after sleep. Sensation as if little hammers were beating in head.

Nux Vomica 30c: Headache with retching, vomiting and often constipation, worse in morning; either at back of head or over one eye.

Cell Salts

Ferr Phos: Headache with bloodshot eyes; often accompanies a cold.

Kali Phos: Headache with bad breath, brown-coated tongue, worse from noise and lack of sleep; child may be nervous, excitable type.

Mag Phos: Headache with eye troubles; sparks before eyes; shooting pains into head.

Nat Mur: Dull, heavy head with watering eyes and constipation.

SEEK MEDICAL, HOMOEOPATHIC OR NATUROPATHIC ADVICE

If headaches are severe, or recur frequently.

See also: Allergy, Eyes – Eyestrain, Influenza, Meningitis, Hepatitis, Measles.

HOW TO USE: HERBS, PAGE 16 | HOMOEOPATHICS, PAGE 20 | CELL SALTS, PAGE 25

Heat Exhaustion/Heat Stroke

A profound failure of the circulation to regulate the temperature level. May be brought on by high atmospheric temperatures; high humidity with low air current; or inability to sweat, poor ventilation, overcrowding, being overdressed (babies or toddlers), high fever (e.g. malaria). Sunstroke can mark the beginning of heatstroke.

DESCRIPTION – Heat Exhaustion

Weakness, faintness, profuse sweating but stable temperature (some children may not sweat); large pupils; pale, cool skin; muscle cramps. Fast shallow breathing; rapid, weak pulse.

WHAT TO DO

Place child at rest in a cool place; elevate legs.
Due to loss of salt and minerals, give Electrolyte solution (or make up $1/2$ tsp salt, 8 tsp sugar/honey in 500 ml/17 fl oz boiled water). Take as frequent small drinks.
Avoid re-exposure to heat.
Watch for shock reaction.

DESCRIPTION – Heatstroke

Vomiting, headache, nausea; red, hot and dry skin – not even armpits are moist; increase in temperature pulse; drowsiness; maybe diarrhoea. In serious cases there may be delirium and eventually unconsciousness. Heatstroke can be very dangerous.

WHAT TO DO

This is an emergency. **SEEK MEDICAL AID**.

Cool the body as rapidly as possible with tepid sponging, or lukewarm bath. Alternatively, wrap body in cold wet sheet and keep wet with ice or sprayed water. Fan continually, keep child upright.

If temperature is over 40°C (104°F), use cold water.

If temperature is over 42°C (107.6°F), use iced water if possible.

Give plenty of small drinks of water or unsweetened juice.

Place at rest in a cool place.

Ensure child does not become overheated during the next few weeks.

FOR BOTH HEAT EXHAUSTION AND HEATSTROKE

Herbs

To help stabilize the temperature levels and provide adequate Vitamins C and E: Lavender, Rosemary, Skullcap and Lemon Balm can be sipped often. These can be taken together or separately.

Homoeopathic

Belladonna 30c: Bounding pulse, delirium, burning red hot and dry skin. Pupils are dilated and fixed.

Bryonia 30c: Splitting headache, worse from sitting up and moving about which make child nauseous.

China 30c: Great exhaustion brought on by excessive sweating; hot face with cold hands.

Cuprum Met 30c: When accompanied by convulsions and severe cramps.

Gelsemium 30c: Worse from exposure to sun; recurrent fever and weakness; tired eyes and limbs, depression.

Glonoine 30c: Surging of blood to head and neck; sees sparks; throbbing headache worse from heat, hot flushed face and sweaty skin.

Mezereum 30c: Give night and morning before exposure, for those who are greatly affected by the heat.

HOW TO USE: HERBS, PAGE 16 | HOMOEOPATHICS, PAGE 20 | CELL SALTS, PAGE 25

Hepatitis

A *notifiable disease:* must be reported to a medical doctor.

An inflammation of the liver which can be caused by a variety of agents such as infections, toxic drugs and poisons.

Hepatitis A is infectious, occurring sporadically or in epidemics; transmitted orally by hand or by flies contaminated by the motions of a person with hepatitis or by dirty water.

Hepatitis B is also infectious. A serum hepatitis, it can be transmitted via blood products or by contact with body fluids of an infected person.

DESCRIPTION – Hepatitis A

Quick onset; gastrointestinal disturbance, fever, lack of appetite, aching in back and limbs, vomiting, diarrhoea, itchy skin, weight loss. Jaundice (yellowing of skin and eyes) appears as other symptoms improve. Depression and tiredness can persist for some months. If symptoms persist for six months or more after an acute attack, this is known as Chronic Hepatitis.

Incubation period: 30–40 days.

Isolation period: Until fever subsides.

Recovery rate: 3–16 weeks.

DESCRIPTION – Hepatitis B

Sudden onset; headache, fever, chills, general weakness, nausea, vomiting, abdominal pains, jaundice. Depression and tiredness can persist for some months. If symptoms persist for six months or more after an acute attack, this is known as Chronic Hepatitis.

Incubation period: 41–108 days.

DESCRIPTION – Hepatitis C

Transmitted by blood contact, constant lower resistance to infection, can cause liver damage in the long term.

WHAT TO DO

The same approach applies to all forms of hepatitis.

Seek medical advice if suspected.

Avoid physical exertion, unnecessary travel, strong medication, wherever possible.

Food is best kept to a bare minimum. Use fresh fruits and vegetables if child is hungry.

Avoid fried foods, fatty foods, egg yolks, excess protein and alcohol.

Beetroot, carrot and dandelion juices are especially beneficial. Freshly squeezed citrus juice mixed with water (1:1) should be sipped daily.

Herbs

To strengthen the liver: Barberry, Mandrake and/or Yarrow, Milk Thistle (helps build new cells), Licorice, Fennel, Dandelion, Burdock.

To restore energy: Gentian.

As antiseptic: Golden Seal or Thyme.

For diarrhoea: Meadowsweet, Raspberry.

For extra nourishment: Lemon and Rosemary.

For depression: Gotu Kola, St Johns Wort.

Homoeopathic

After suspected contact, see Resistance and Immunity, page 29.

Bryonia 30c: Child is irritable, nauseous and dizzy. Liver is swollen with stitching pain in upper right side of abdomen and under right shoulder blade: bitter taste in mouth. Child is worse from motion, better lying on right side.

Chelidonium 30c: Sore, stitching pain in liver; pain under liver and lower angle of right shoulder blade; fever, chills and diarrhoea.

China 30c: Shooting, pressing pain in liver; liver feels swollen and hard; tongue has thick, yellow coating with bitter taste.

Hepar Sulph 30c: Irritable; heaviness and pressure after slight meal, stitching in liver worse from walking, laughing, breathing, pressure.

HOW TO USE: HERBS, PAGE 16 | HOMOEOPATHICS, PAGE 20 | CELL SALTS, PAGE 25

Mercurius 30c: Liver swollen and sore to touch; stabbing pain, cannot lie on right side; teeth imprints on yellow tongue; foul breath.

Nat Sulph 30c: Bursting feeling in head with burning in stomach; vomiting of bile; aching, cutting pain in liver, yellow complexion and eyes, cannot bear anything tight around waist; worse lying on left side.

Cell Salts

Kali Mur: Jaundice with constipation, swollen liver, white-coated tongue, lack of appetite, light-coloured stools and headache.

Nat Sulph: Liver is sore, congested; child is yellow, vomits bile and has a greenish coating on tongue.

LONG-TERM APPROACH

If child continues to remain tired and depressed after hepatitis, continue with above herbs and dietary recommendations daily.

Calc Phos 6x can be very helpful if child develops symptoms of twitching, jerking, itching and weakness. Give twice daily for several weeks.

TO BUILD RESISTANCE

To help strengthen the immune system and restore to full health after disease or vaccination, see page 29.

Hives

Hives (Urticaria) may follow stings, insect bites or trauma. They may also be due to sensitivity to certain foods or drugs, e.g. shellfish, strawberries, eggs, chocolate, penicillin or antibiotics.

Hives may also be associated with worm infestations.

DESCRIPTION

Extremely itchy, red spots which can be any size or shape, over a large part of the body especially the mouth and throat. These spots may become swollen and slightly elevated. Hives fade quickly only to reappear elsewhere.

WHAT TO DO

Herbs

To bathe and soothe the affected parts: Dandelion, Yarrow and Golden Seal, can also be taken internally.

Homoeopathic

Antim Crud 6c: Burning and itching skin, worse from warmth and heat of bed, worse on cheeks and chin.

Camphor 6c: Hives from eating shellfish, usually erysipelas.

Candida 6c: When rash appears after penicillin or antibiotics (or urtica urens).

Pulsatilla 6c: Worse after eating rich foods, often with diarrhoea.

Rhus Tox 6c: Swollen rash with numerous spots; great itching and tingling.

Urtica Urens 6c: Burning, stinging rash. Intolerable itching. Worse after eating shellfish. This is the most commonly used remedy.

Cell Salts

Kali Phos: Hives caused by food.

Nat Mur: Hives caused by insect bites.

HOW TO USE: HERBS, PAGE 16 | HOMOEOPATHICS, PAGE 20 | CELL SALTS, PAGE 25

Nat Phos: Hives that appear when worms are suspected.

External application:
Cell salts can be applied locally to the hives by crushing 3–4 tablets
and mixing with $1/2$ cup of water.

Impetigo/School Sores

A contagious infection of the superficial layers of the skin, maybe due to a streptococcal or staphylococcal infection.

DESCRIPTION

Starts as red spots on normal skin (usually around nose and mouth). These progress from watery-looking blisters to pus-filled sores which rupture, discharge and spread. The broken blisters leave raw skin which then forms a crust.

In babies the impetigo usually develops in areas such as the armpit or groin, and in older children it usually starts on the face near the mouth, nose or ears.

Impetigo can follow a cold.

It can spread rapidly by direct contact.

It is more common in warm weather.

WHAT TO DO

Do not let child touch spots as this spreads infection.

Herbs

Dab infected sores with alcohol (vodka is satisfactory). This helps to clean and dry out the sores, although it does sting for a moment.

Remove any soft crusts and apply Calendula Ointment often.

Alternatively, Oils of Teatree or Thyme can be applied, directly or diluted (2 drops to 3 tsps Olive or Soya Oil).

Internally:
To purify the blood: Drink Dandelion, Echinacea or Red Clover.
As antiseptic: Golden Seal.
To soothe from the inside out: Slippery Elm.

HOW TO USE: HERBS, PAGE 16 | HOMOEOPATHICS, PAGE 20 | CELL SALTS, PAGE 25

Homoeopathic

See Remedy Pictures (page 199) for constitutional type.

Antim Crud 30c: Thick, yellow, spreading crusts; thick, white-coated tongue; worse from bathing.

Arsen Alb 30c: Thin, watery discharge which burns and reddens the skin.

Calc Carb 30c: Eruption oozes a thick, bland discharge. Useful during teething.

Hepar Sulph 30c: Soft crusts with thin, yellow pus; sore and bleeding easily; very red and sensitive to touch; worse from cold air, and cold bathing.

Mercurius 30c: Sores affect the deeper skin layers; look ulcerated and bleed.

Rhus Tox 30c: Eruptions in clusters; dark-coloured discharge with violent burning and itching, tingling and stinging.

Strep/Staph 30c: For recurring impetigo or no reaction to well-chosen remedies.

Influenza

A highly infectious disease caused by a number of viruses affecting the upper respiratory tract and the body, acting more widely than the common cold virus.

DESCRIPTION

Begins as a headache, fever (highest on the second day 38–40.5°C (100.4–105°F) with sore throat, severe pain in limbs and back. After a few days there is more debilitation with running nose and cough, leaving child depressed, exhausted, uncomfortable and weary.

Incubation Period: 2–3 days.

Recovery Time: 3–7 days if no complications arise.

Complications: Can arise from lack of attention to the recuperation period when depression, palpitations and broncho-pneumonia can develop.

WHAT TO DO

Rest until temperature returns to normal.

Plenty of diluted pure fruit juices for a few days to rest the digestive organs.

Avoid food during acute phase. If especially hungry, then give fresh fruit, slowly adding vegetables and avoiding dairy foods, processed foods, breads and meats.

Herbs

For fever: Boneset, Yarrow or Lemon Balm.

To soothe and calm: Elder.

To relieve congestion: Echinacea, Garlic, Golden Seal, Cayenne, Ginger.

For disturbed digestion: Cinnamon or Thyme.

Externally: Peppermint or Teatree Oil (3 drops diluted with 2 tsp Olive Oil) can be used as a rub on the sore parts.

HOW TO USE: HERBS, PAGE 16 | HOMOEOPATHICS, PAGE 20 | CELL SALTS, PAGE 25

Homoeopathic

After suspected contact, see Resistance and Immunity, page 29.

Arsen Alb 30c: Can't bear sight or smell of food; sneezing, thin watery discharge; dry cough; painful chest; burning eyes.

Baptisia 30c: Sore muscles, offensive breath, stool, urine and/or sweat; sense of suffocation in chest.

Eupatorium Perfoliatum 30c: Great soreness and aching all over body; sore larynx and chest; child holds chest during cough because it hurts so much; also pain in head during cough; runny nose and great thirst.

Euphrasia 30c: If the eyes are very much affected.

Gelsemium 30c: Aching limbs; dull, heavy eyes and head; child is weak, tired and chilly; bouts of sneezing.

Phosphorus 30c: For debility following influenza.

Pyrogenium 30c: Restless, rapid pulse, sweat but no heat; bed feels too hard.

Rhus Tox 30c: Caused by getting wet and cold; sneezing, bone pains and depression.

Influenzinum or Bacillinum 30c (Nosode – see page 31): To help clear a severe case or for lingering after-effects of the disease.

TO BUILD RESISTANCE

To help strengthen the immune system and restore to full health after the disease or vaccination, see page 29.

See also: Cold, Cough, Allergy, Throat (Sore), Bronchitis (Influenza fever is normally higher than Bronchitis).

Jaundice

Jaundice is the term given to the yellow discoloration of the skin and conjunctiva (inside eyelid) caused by an excess of bile pigment in the bloodstream. This yellowish colour is the indicating symptom.

Types of Jaundice
The abnormal presence of bile in the blood may be caused by:

1. Blockage or interference in the bile ducts (Obstructive or Cholestatic Jaundice): Caused by gallstones, drugs, recurrent jaundice in pregnancy or viral hepatitis (*see* Hepatitis).
   Signs may be: Pale stools, dark urine, great weight loss, persistent itching, painful enlarged spleen, enlarged neck glands, cholesterol deposits around eyelids.
2. A disorder of liver function (Hepatocellular, Infective or Toxic Jaundice): The liver cells cannot excrete bilirubin into bile duct for excretion.
   Caused by: Viral infection transmitted by droplets from mouth or nose; yellow fever; drugs or toxic agents such as phosphorus, arsenic, gold or chloroform.
   In babies, it may be due to an umbilical infection; in older children it is usually brought about by chemicals.
   After an incubation period of 4–5 weeks, symptoms of gastric disturbance with vomiting persist for many weeks.
3. Excessive destruction of red blood cells (Haemolytic or Physiological Jaundice): Occurring within the first few days of life, it is seldom a serious problem now. (When due to Rh Factor incompatibility, the infant will be kept in hospital and may need a transfusion. This is rare since 1975.)
   Caused by: Breakdown of red blood cells present in the newborn as the lung functions take over from the placenta.
   Signs: Yellow discoloration of skin and other tissues (not eyes); bowel motions retain their normal colour; this type of jaundice passes off after two weeks without complications.

HOW TO USE: HERBS, PAGE 16 | HOMOEOPATHICS, PAGE 20 | CELL SALTS, PAGE 25

WHAT TO DO

SEEK MEDICAL ADVICE

The cause needs to be identified and jaundice due to viruses is a *notifiable disease* (the Department of Health must be informed to alert contacts).

Also, seek advice from a natural health practitioner.

Any treatment can be supported by the following:

Bed rest in a well-ventilated room.

In Infectious Jaundice, avoid contact with others.

In jaundice of the newborn baby, place a few drops of wheat germ oil in a dropper into the mouth once daily until yellowness fades. Expose child's skin to sunlight gently.

Light nourishing diet, avoid fats, fried food, alcohol and roast foods.

Drink plenty of fluids: skimmed milk, juices made from lemon, carrot, apple, beetroot, celery and grapes mixed with honey if desired and taken several times daily for months. Raw apples, pears and grapes.

Barley Water (1 cup barley simmered with 3 litres/5 pints water for 3 hours and strained).

Herbs

Many herbs are of benefit to the liver during jaundice and convalescence. Mix any combination of the following and drink small glasses 3–4 times daily: Dandelion, Centaury, Irish Moss, Agrimony, Rosehip, Barberry, Blue Flag, Yellow Dock, Golden Seal, Mandrake, Cascara Sagrada.

Homoeopathic

Aconite 30c: Fever, restlessness, anxiety, pressure and constriction around liver; white stools; alternately loose stools and constipation.

Arsen Alb 30c: Great exhaustion after slight exertion; low vitality; great thirst; no appetite; vomiting of blood and bile; belching;

very irritable stomach, swollen painful liver and spleen, burning pain in rectum and anus. Itchy skin. Disturbed restless sleep.

Chelidonium 30c: For jaundiced babies in first few weeks of life, half crushed tablet or one drop daily till jaundice fades. Biliousness and jaundice, swelling of liver, chilliness, fever, yellow-coated tongue, bitter taste and craving for acid things; stools yellow, profuse and loose.

China 30c: Exhaustion from longstanding jaundice; white stools with flatulence; stools soft but difficult to pass; swollen liver and spleen; disturbed anxious sleep; thickly coated dirty tongue.

Hydrastis 30c: Bitter taste, lack of appetite, yellow smelly urine, exhaustion, light-coloured stools; slimy, swollen, white tongue. Tender liver, constipation.

Merc Corr 30c: Yellow, white-coated tongue with teeth imprints, foul breath, lost appetite; depressed and low-spirited; clay-coloured stools with much straining to pass them; yellow skin over eyes; liver region painful to touch; itching all over.

Merc Dulcis 30c: Jaundice in children with offensive breath; nausea and vomiting; dark tongue; bowel motion with bile, mucous and blood.

Phosphorus 30c: Marked soreness of liver with jaundice; depressed, easily startled; nervous; greyish-white stools; vomiting; painless, copious debilitating diarrhoea, dark urine with sediment; great drowsiness; short naps and frequent wakings. Worse from exertion.

Podophyllum 30c: Alternate diarrhoea and constipation; loose and watery or hard and clay-coloured stool; yellow face and eyes; vomiting; hot, sour belching; foul taste; liver painful worse from rubbing; pain under right shoulder blade; white or yellow-coated tongue. Maybe gallstones.

Sulphur 30c: Chronic jaundice though not indicated if stools are colourless. Irritable, depressed, thin and weak with good appetite; itchy skin; sore and red anus; morning diarrhoea; wakens suddenly.

Note: Cholesterinum 6x: three times daily for 2–4 weeks taken with your choice of above, for burning pain in side, gallstones, hurts so much, holds hands on sides.

HOW TO USE: HERBS, PAGE 16 | HOMOEOPATHICS, PAGE 20 | CELL SALTS, PAGE 25

Cell Salts

Ferr Phos: For pain in liver with vomiting of undigested food.

Kali Mur: Jaundice with catarrhal condition; constipation; light-coloured stools.

Kali Sulph: Slimy-yellow coating on tongue, catarrh of stomach; fullness at pit of stomach.

Nat Mur: Jaundice associated with drowsiness, watery secretions, thirst, dryness of skin.

Measles

An infectious disease
A highly contagious viral infection transferred by droplets from the mouth or nose when child coughs, talks or sneezes.

DESCRIPTION

Begins with cold symptoms – running nose, sore throat, cough, red watery eyes, often a dislike of bright light and a fever that becomes progressively higher (up to 40.5°C/105°F). About four days later a rash of red-pink blotches appear – first behind the ears and on the face, sometimes inside the mouth, and spreading to trunk and limbs.

The fever should subside at this stage.

After another 5–7 days the rash begins to fade.

The fever accompanying measles can become very high, and the appetite may be completely lost.

Most common age: 8 months to 5 years.

Incubation period: 10–14 days.

Isolation period: 1 week after rash appears.

Recovery time: A mild attack is over well within a fortnight.

Complications: Secondary infection of middle ear, throat, larynx or lungs; encephalitis; visual disturbances.

WHAT TO DO

- Put to bed and avoid bright lights; keep out those visitors who have colds and sore throats; have room quiet and warm; avoid use of eyes, e.g. reading or watching television.
- Drink *lots* of fluids; if child has no appetite, he/she will receive adequate nourishment from herb teas and diluted fruit or vegetable juices during the acute stage of the illness.
- If earache develops, seek professional advice from your doctor or homoeopath.
- **SEEK MEDICAL ADVICE** if signs of pneumonia, meningitis, severe tummy pain develop.

HOW TO USE: HERBS, PAGE 16 | HOMOEOPATHICS, PAGE 20 | CELL SALTS, PAGE 25

Herbs

To move the bowels: Liquorice.

For fever: Boneset.

To calm and soothe the system: Hops or Elder.

To ease the rash: Red Clover.

For cough: Mullein.

For restoring energy: Gentian.

To provide extra nourishment during illness: Lavender, Teatree or Thyme.

Inhalation: Oils of Lavender (3 drops), Teatree (2 drops) and Thyme (1 drop) mixed with steaming water (1 litre/1^3/$_4$ pints) can be breathed in to help the nose and eyes.

External: Thyme Oil (3 drops) can be mixed with Olive or Soya Oil (2 tsp) and rubbed on rash to soothe.

Homoeopathic

After suspected contact see Resistance and Immunity, page 29.

Apis 30c: High temperature, very hot and wanting covers off, sore eyes, tearful and irritable.

Bryonia 30c: Tiresome cough. High temperature, swollen face with dull look, complains of headache, intense thirst for cold water, feels chilly but wants air. Dry, hard, painful cough; appearance of rash is delayed.

Euphrasia 30c: Red, swollen eyelids and great sensitivity to light.

Gelsemium 30c: Very high fever, limbs feel too heavy to move; maybe delirium. Harsh, barking cough with sore chest and dislike of company. Absence of thirst with dry tongue; red, itchy skin.

Phosphorus 30c: Chest symptoms prominent; troublesome dry cough and tightness in chest; thirst for cold water which may be vomited.

Pulsatilla 30c: Useful after fever stage. Very restless and irritable, wants to be constantly waited on; child must sit up with troublesome cough, loose by day and dry by night; maybe nausea, diarrhoea or earache.

Morbillinum 30c (Nosode – see page 31). To help clear a severe case or for lingering after-effects of the disease. Do not give whilst disease is incubating.

Cell Salts

Ferr Phos: First remedy for fever and until eruption appears.

Kali Mur: Coated tongue, ear problems, swollen glands and hoarse cough.

Nat Mur: Very itchy skin and watery nose and eyes.

Give the appropriate cell salt hourly until the eruption appears. They may be alternated if necessary.

Alternate Calc Phos and Kali Sulph during the final stages to help clear the condition and restore energy.

TO BUILD RESISTANCE

To help strengthen the immune system and restore to full health after the disease (or vaccination), see page 29.

SEEK MEDICAL ADVICE

If child develops:

Shortness of breath with the cough.

Earache or swollen glands.

Convulsions.

Headache and vomiting.

Lethargy and lack of awareness of surroundings.

Eyes become stuck together and very red.

Fever *remains* two days after the spots appear.

Severe tummy pain.

See also: Rubella, Scarlet Fever, Bronchitis, Influenza.

HOW TO USE: HERBS, PAGE 16 | HOMOEOPATHICS, PAGE 20 | CELL SALTS, PAGE 25

Meningitis

A notifiable disease: Must be reported immediately.
Inflammation of the meninges (brain lining) caused by bacterial, chemical, fungal or viral invasion.
Meningitis can be epidemic or follow an infection e.g. respiratory, middle ear or sinus.

DESCRIPTION

Some or all of the following may occur:

Fever and stiff neck, headache, irritable and drowsy; can deteriorate to include convulsions, delirium and respiratory difficulties.
Incubation period: 3–7 days.
Isolation period: until cured.
Complications: hydrocephalus, nerve palsy, renal failure.

WHAT TO DO

Seek medical advice immediately (Successful recovery depends on speed of treatment. Child will be admitted to hospital for lumbar puncture and blood tests and probably get intravenous antibiotics.)

The following procedure is included for your information to aid in restoring to full health after medical treatment *or* until medical aid arrives. Take child off all foods and give a diet of fresh fruit juices and vegetable juices, herb teas and broths.

Herbs
Combine any of the following:

To calm the nervous system: Skullcap or Valerian.
To fight the infection: Golden Seal.
To reduce fever: Yarrow.
To provide extra nourishment during the illness: Peppermint and Rosemary.

Homoeopathic

After suspected contact, see Resistance and Immunity, page 29.

Aconite 30c: Useful at beginning when fear is marked. If symptoms come on after exposure to the sun.

Apis 30c: Shrill outcries in sleep; fidgety; violent fever, swelling and grinding of teeth.

Belladonna 30c: Burning fever; throat spasm worse from swallowing; uncontrollable vomiting; bluish-red facial colour; dilated eyes; headache worse from light noise and jarring. Starts in sleep and grinds teeth. Violent symptom.

Bryonia 30c: Chewing motion of mouth; screams in pain if moved; distended abdomen; copious sweat; drinks in greedy fashion. Face flushes and pales alternately. White tongue.

Calc Carb 30c: Large-headed children; pale face; large abdomen; sweaty head worse during sleep; screaming without cause, strong urine.

Cuprum 30c: Excessive vomiting, worse from movement or touch; convulsions with blue face and contracted jaws; craves cold water. Violent delirium, rolling eyeballs, deep sleep.

Helleborus 30c: Unconscious moaning, rolling head, dropping jaw; foul smell; cannot be fully aroused; wrinkling of forehead; automatic movements of one arm and leg. Eyeballs turned upwards, shooting pains in head, bores head into pillow.

Stramonium 30c: Convulsions of upper extremities and isolated muscles; staggering, stammering, vomiting green bile; terrified expression; cannot swallow because of spasm.

Zincum 30c: Sharp pains in head; fidgety feet; little or no fever. Hypersensitivity of skin and senses.

Meningococcin 30c (Nosode – see page 31): To help clear a severe case or for lingering after-effects of the disease. *Do not give whilst disease is incubating.*

Cell Salts

All of the following are needed:

Ferr Phos and Kali Phos to be alternated every half hour.

Nat Mur: Give this also at two-hourly intervals.

Silica: Give this once daily.

HOW TO USE: HERBS, PAGE 16 | HOMOEOPATHICS, PAGE 20 | CELL SALTS, PAGE 25

TO BUILD RESISTANCE

To help strengthen the immune system, restore to full health after the disease (or vaccination), see Resistance and Immunity, page 29.

Menstruation

The appearance of the first menstrual period varies from age 9–18, but is most common between ages 12–14.

For some girls approaching their teenage years, the hormonal changes can cause major discomfort in the form of mood changes, period pains, heavy or irregular periods, headaches, fevers, nausea, dizziness or vomiting.

These symptoms can serve a useful purpose by showing us the constitutional tendencies of the person concerned. Homoeopathy and herbs have much to offer for this issue. We feel that by dealing with these crises when they first occur, many potential adult problems can be avoided.

WHAT TO DO

The remedies below may not offer a solution for every young woman, in which case we recommend that you seek expert herbal or homoeopathic advice.

For the emotional problems associated with hormonal changes, Bach Flower Essences have much to offer. Related books and remedies are available from most health shops.

Herbs

For an irregular cycle or absent period (unless pregnancy is suspected): Blue Cohosh, False Unicorn Rt, Sabina, Rue, Southernwood, Tansy, Pennyroyal, Parsley, Senecio, Motherwort, Black Cohosh, Blessed Thistle or Vitex Agnus Castus.

Heavy flow: Ladies Mantle, Plantain, Comfrey, Mistletoe, Blessed Thistle, Yarrow, Don Quai.

Painful cramps: Cramp Bark, Passionflower, Black Cohosh, False Unicorn Root, Wild Yam, Dandelion, Chamomile.

Premenstrual tension: Skullcap, Valerian, Chamomile, Bach Flower Essences.

HOW TO USE: HERBS, PAGE 16 | HOMOEOPATHICS, PAGE 20 | CELL SALTS, PAGE 25

Homoeopathy

Aconite 30c: Period suppressed due to chill or fright; headache with apprehension and restlessness. Worse from heat. Thirsty with red face.

Belladonna 30c: Irregular and profuse. Face red and flushed, thirsty, restless and irritable. Cutting pains.

Bryonia 30c: Irregular or suppressed period with headache or nose-bleed, and constipation.

Calc Carb 30c: First period begins very early. Sluggish, overweight and pale; itchy genitals before period with tender, swollen breasts. Headache, colic, chilliness and sweat are common before the period.

Chamomilla 30c: Severe colicky pains, restless and irritable, diarrhoea and fainting.

Ferr Met 30c: Thin, tired, anaemic girl with irregular period of pale watery blood.

Graphites 30c: Very late first period. Irregular period with constipation, itching of genitals, swollen, hard breasts, and skin problems.

Ignatia 30c: Period is affected by grief or shock.

Kali Carb 30c: Delayed and difficult first period in young girls accompanied by fear and anxiety and pain through back, abdomen and genitals.

Nat Mur 30c: Early, heavy period in a weepy, emotional girl with shiny facial skin.

Nux Vomica 30c: Painful cramps and violent spasms, irritable and constipated.

Pulsatilla 30c: First period is delayed, slight loss only, with back pain, nausea, crying, vomiting. Period is changeable, may stop suddenly after exposure to dampness or wet.

Sepia 30c: Depressed, irritable and solitary girl; thin, tired, sallow-coloured skin, dragging down pains in abdomen; frequently delayed period.

Sulphur 30c: Untidy, disorganized person. Hot, burning period pains; red face, blood nose, irregular period stopping suddenly or preceded by headache.

Cell Salts

Calc Phos: Scanty flow, difficult first periods, anaemic with colicky pains and backache.

Ferr Phos: Painful period preceded by congestion in pelvic organs and headache. Flushing, fever and vomiting.

Kali Mur: Painful period worse from taking cold; blood is a very dark colour.

Kali Phos: Menstrual colic in pale, tearful, irritable, sensitive, nervous girls.

Mag Phos: Spasms of cramp-like pain in lower abdomen causing her to bend over double; better from heat and movement.

Nat Mur: Irregular period, scanty and dark, preceded by frontal headache, flow is irritating; girl is depressed and withdrawn.

Silica: Icy coldness of entire body before and during period with constipation, anxiety and oversensitive nature.

HOW TO USE: HERBS, PAGE 16 | HOMOEOPATHICS, PAGE 20 | CELL SALTS, PAGE 25

Mouth Ulcers

Recurrent, painful mouth sores.
If one or more sores causes bleeding when scraped, thrush is suspected. Cracks at corners of mouth indicate Vitamin B2 or B3 deficiency. Nuts, chocolates and citrus fruits can cause recurrence of mouth ulcers; ulcers may also be caused by bowel inflammation or physical and emotional stress.

WHAT TO DO

Herbs

Gargle and also use as herbal tea one or more of the following herbs; Myrrh, Golden Seal, Raspberry, Marjoram or Sage.
Teatree Oil may be applied directly to the ulcer.

Homoeopathic

Borax 30c: Small ulcers that bleed if touched, or when eating; mouth is hot.
Mercurius 30c: Much saliva with spongy gums, sweet metallic taste and thirst.
Nitric Acid 30c: Ulcers with splinter-like pains, bad breath and much saliva. Whitish gums.

Cell Salts

Calc Phos: Blisters on tip of tongue; cold sores or chapped lips.
Kali Mur: Rawness of mouth.
Nat Mur: Blisters on tongue.
Silica: Ulcers on tongue.

See also: Thrush, Cold Sores.

Mumps

An infectious disease.
A viral infection of one or both parotid glands.
The virus spreads by means of droplets from the mouth or nose while coughing, talking or sneezing.

DESCRIPTION

Begins with nasal catarrh, a rise in temperature (37.5–39.5°C/99.5–103°F), a mild feeling of illness, and tenderness around the ears, followed by swelling of the parotid gland (situated immediately in front of the ear lobes and at the angle of the jaw). The other parotid usually swells a day or two later. There is pain on chewing and opening mouth and the outline of the face is altered considerably.

Note: Swelling is particularly in front, below and behind the ear lobe and when swollen, is hard, tense and immovable.

If there is any doubt, seek further advice in order to distinguish from the more serious diphtheria. (However, this is no longer common.)

Most common age: 5 to 15 years.

Incubation period: 18 days.

Isolation period: For 9 days from the date of onset or until swelling of all involved glands has completely subsided and the patient has returned to normal.

Recovery time: 7–10 days.

WHAT TO DO

Rest and warmth; restricted diet of fresh fruits, vegetables, soups, broths and fresh juices.

Herbs

To clear out the lymph glands: Daily drinks of Red Clover Tea during the mumps and afterwards.

To keep bowels clear: Drink Liquorice and Rosemary Tea.

HOW TO USE: HERBS, PAGE 16 | HOMOEOPATHICS, PAGE 20 | CELL SALTS, PAGE 25

Homoeopathic

After suspected contact: Pilocarpine 30c. This can help the child's resistance to the disease. Give one dose night and morning for three days (starting within 2 days of contact) then one dose per week for 2 weeks.

Belladonna 30c: Bright red swelling on right side; also useful where swelling disappears and head or neck pain develops.

Bryonia 30c: Hard swelling with tenderness; slightest motion of head is painful; irritable; dry lips; very thirsty for large quantities of water.

Mercurius 30c: For slight fever with tenderness in neck area; excess saliva and offensive breath; much pain and stiffness in jaws.

Pulsatilla 30c: If disease lingers, weepy, whining, thirstless child who craves the open air.

Rhus Tox 30c: Dark, red swellings; sticking pains on swallowing; worse left side.

Parotidinum 30c (Nosode – see page 31): To help clear a severe case, or for lingering after-effects of the disease. *Do not give whilst disease is incubating.*

Cell Salts

Calc Fluor: If swelling persists past expected duration.

Ferr Phos: For early stage of fever and pain.

Kali Mur and Nat Mur: Alternate when gland is swollen and painful with thickly-coated white tongue.

SEEK MEDICAL ADVICE

If the child develops a bad headache, vomiting, neck stiffness or drowsiness.

If boys of eleven years or older develop swelling and pain in the testicles.

If girls of eleven years or older develop breast pains.

If any other glands are swollen.

TO BUILD RESISTANCE

To strengthen the immune system and help restore to full health after the disease or vaccination, see Resistance and Immunity, page 29.

Nappy Rash

Seen as sore, red, scalded skin on bottom and nappy area.

WHAT TO DO

Rinse nappies thoroughly in 1 tbsp vinegar per $1/2$ litre (17 fl oz) of water. Be aware that, in some cases, disposable nappies can aggravate nappy rash. Expose skin to air a few hours every day. Do not leave wet nappies on.

Long-continuing or severe nappy rash may be an indication of a more serious skin condition, such as eczema or psoriasis.

Herbs

Any of the following may be helpful when applied locally to the rash: Calendula Ointment, Apricot Kernel or Avocado Oil, Aloe Vera Gel.

Homoeopathic

Borax 30c: Rash between thighs in babies subject to thrush.

Calc Carb 30c: In babies who perspire easily with cold hands and feet; eruptions may be pustular or scaly-looking; itching, smarting, worse from cold.

Graphites 30c: Skin harsh, dry, thickened, rough and easily chafed. Better from warmth and dryness. Usually accompanied by constipation.

Hepar Sulph 30c: Genital area inflamed and itching; very sensitive when exposed to cold air, touch, undressing. Better from warmth.

Sulphur 30c: Dry, itchy, scaly, red eruption on genital area. Worse at night, and in bed.

External application: Urtica Urens Cream or Tincture (10 drops to $1/2$ glass water).

Cell Salts

Nat Phos: Counteracts too much acidity.

Nat Mur: For chafed skin.

Crush 3 tablets of either cell salt, mix with 1 tbsp water and apply to the rash.

HOW TO USE: HERBS, PAGE 16 | HOMOEOPATHICS, PAGE 20 | CELL SALTS, PAGE 25

Nose

1 Congestion
2 Nosebleed
3 Object in the nose

1 Congestion

Congestion can involve a blocked nose, a free-flowing discharge, or a thick, yellow discharge (which often indicates infection).
It can also coincide with influenza, measles, colds or allergies. *See also* Sinusitis.

WHAT TO DO

Herbs

To dry up mucous: Yarrow.
To cleanse: Thyme.
To soothe the mucous membranes: Slippery Elm.
For Vitamin C: Rosehip.
To provide extra nourishment: Clove, Aniseed or Thyme.
   Mix any of these together and drink warm throughout the day.
Inhalation to clear nostrils: 3–8 drops of Thyme, Peppermint or Teatree Oil into a basin of steaming water. Place head over basin, cover head with towel and breathe in the vapour for ten minutes. Repeat as required.

Homoeopathic

Aconite 30c: Nose is swollen, dry or blocked with tingling, burning and throbbing sensations. Worse from cold, dry winds, better in open air.
Arsen Alb 30c: Thin, watery discharge which burns the skin; intense tickling; nose feels blocked. Chilliness, sneezing. Worse in open air.
Gelsemium 30c: Sneezing, runny nose with heavy eyes, fullness at root of nose, headache; child is worse in warm weather.

Hepar Sulph 30c: Nose is blocked in cold air; discharge becomes thick, yellow; nose is painful and swollen; child is irritable. Easy recurrence accompanied by sticking in throat.

Mercurius 30c: Nostrils are raw and ulcerated with thin mucous, burning in eyes and nose; frontal sinus involvement.

Nat Mur 30c: For colds beginning with a sneeze; watery, clear discharge; loss of smell and taste. Blisters around mouth and nose.

Nux Vomica 30c: Nose is alternately dry and fluent in the daytime, blocked at night and outdoors.

Pulsatilla 30c: Thick, yellow, bland discharge; loss of taste, smell and appetite; better in the cool air; worse from warmth.

Cell Salts

Calc Phos: Swollen, ulcerated nostrils; icy cold tip of nose; child takes cold easily.

Kali Mur: Discharge drops down back of throat; or is thick and white.

Kali Sulph: Yellow, slimy discharge.

Nat Mur: Thin, salty, watery discharge; sneezing.

Nat Sulph: Discharge is either green and profuse or dry and burning.

Silica: Nostrils are either red and sore or itchy and dry.

FOR RECURRING CONGESTION

Refer Allergies if nasal congestion often recurs. Incompletely cleared infections may contribute to nasal congestion.

Herbs

Rosehip, Echinacea, Golden Seal and Mullein can be taken daily for several weeks. These are rich in Vitamins A and C which help fight infection.

2 Nosebleed

Sit child up, leaning forward with a pad to collect blood. Squeeze the soft part of the nose at nostrils for ten minutes by the clock.

HOW TO USE: HERBS, PAGE 16 | HOMOEOPATHICS, PAGE 20 | CELL SALTS, PAGE 25

Release and observe – if bleeding continues, repeat. Don't let child blow his/her nose for several hours.

Externally: Cold water or ice can be applied to the root of the nose to stop bleeding.

Herbs

Yarrow or Plantain tea sipped at 15-minute intervals.

Hamemelis Tincture (10 drops in $1/2$ cup water) can be used as nose drops (1 drop to each nostril at 5-minute intervals), and can also be taken internally (5 drops at 15-minute intervals).

Homoeopathic

Aconite 30c: Bright, red-coloured blood; child may be anxious or feverish.

Arnica 30c: If bleeding is result of injury.

Hamemelis 30c: Profuse bleeding from nose, non-coagulating flow.

Arsen Album 30c: For recurrent nosebleeds with burning pains and irritability.

China 30c: Easy bleeding from nose, worse after rising and after heavy blowing of nose. Paleness, fainting in anaemic children.

Millefolium 30c: Bright red discharge, maybe after injury. No anxiety.

Phos 30c: Use this first in any case of nosebleed that isn't due to injury.

Cell Salts

Mix Ferr Phos and Kali Mur, three tablets of each mixed in a cup of water and sipped every few minutes during nosebleed.

If tendency is common, take these cell salts twice daily for three weeks.

3 Object in the nose

Child may have difficulty breathing through nose; nose may appear swollen, blood-stained discharge may be seen.

SEEK MEDICAL OR HOSPITAL AID

If object is sharp. Do not attempt to remove the object as it may cause damage to nasal tissues. Advise child to breathe through mouth in the meantime.

If object is hard or spherical (e.g. a marble) as it may go in further. There is then danger of the object going into the lungs or blocking the airways. Advise child to breathe through mouth and do not attempt to remove object.

If object is visible and soft, have child blow out blocked side twice. If it doesn't come out, seek medical or hospital aid.

HOW TO USE: HERBS, PAGE 16 | HOMOEOPATHICS, PAGE 20 | CELL SALTS, PAGE 25

Pneumonia

Pneumonia is an inflammation of the lung, caused by invasion of the pneumonia germ or other germs or viruses. Fluid fills up the lung spaces, making oxygenation less efficient.

DESCRIPTION

Usually starts as a cold with a high fever (39.5–41°C/103–105°F), chills, nausea, severe pain in chest usually on one side, coughing up rusty-coloured, yellow or greenish mucous.

Rapid, shallow breathing; face or fingertips become blue from lack of oxygen; tongue is furred. (Do not confuse with rapid *deep* breathing of dehydration or hyperventilation.)

WHAT TO DO

Seek medical advice immediately
Most children with pneumonia will need antibiotics. The following procedures can be used until medical aid arrives or to help restore child to full health *after medical treatment*.

To aid recovery:
- Plenty of fluid in the form of fresh fruit or vegetable juices, water, or broths. Avoid dairy foods, wheaten products, all forms of sugar and sweetened products.
- Inhalation Oils of Lemon, Lavender, Teatree or Juniper (1 drop of each is usually sufficient) can be added to steaming water and breathed in.

Herbs
Make a mixture from the following:
To ease chest pain: Marshmallow or Mullein.
To cleanse and purify blood: Golden Seal or Garlic.
To move the bowels and thus help eliminate toxins: Liquorice or Rosemary.
To provide extra nourishment during the illness: Lemon, Lavender, Teatree and/or Juniper.

External applications to the chest are very soothing, especially to help through the night. Slightly warm the following mixture and rub onto chest at night and during the day if needed: 2 drops each of Lavender, Lemon, Juniper and Teatree (or Eucalyptus) Oils mixed with 2 tbsp Olive, Soya or Almond Oil.

Homoeopathic

Aconite 30c: Early stage for strong children in whom the attack is sudden; due to cold, dry winds; high sudden fever, hoarse dry cough, short breath, anxiety, palpitations; frothy, watery or blood-tinged sputum; very restless.

Antim Tart 30c: Difficult breathing, worse towards morning, worse from lying down; sharp, burning pains with high fever and occasional vomiting; difficult to raise mucous despite great rattling on chest.

Bryonia 30c: Child lies quietly, cough is dry and painful with scanty rust-coloured sputum. Better from lying on painful or right side, and from keeping still. Child holds breath for fear of cough being too painful.

Iodum 30c: Restlessness with high fever, great difficulty in breathing; blood-streaked sputum, internal heat whilst externally cold. There may be no pain.

Phosphorus 30c: Pneumonia may come on after Measles; hot, tight, painful chest; rattling of mucous with yellow, rusty or blood-streaked sputum. Whole body trembles with the cough. Child is better with sleep and darkness. Feeling of a great load on chest.

Sulphur 30c: Rattling in chest, thick yellow/green sputum, dry tongue, fever; no improvement from other remedies.

Pneumococcin 30c (Nosode – see page 31): To help clear a severe case or for lingering after-effects of the disease. *Do not give whilst disease is incubating.*

Cell Salts

Ferr Phos: During initial stages of infection; short, painful cough; hot chest.

Kali Mur: Thick, white expectoration. Rattling chest.

Kali Sulph: Yellow, slimy, sticky or green mucous; great rattling and wheezing, better in cool air.

HOW TO USE: HERBS, PAGE 16 | HOMOEOPATHICS, PAGE 20 | CELL SALTS, PAGE 25

LONG-TERM

- Depending on the type of Pneumonia, specific Homoeopathic Nosodes are available to help clear residual poisons and restore to full health. Particular homoeopathic remedies that may be found useful are Streptococcin, Influenzinum, Bacillinum and Pneumococcin. Seek homoeopathic advice for use of these.
- After such a debilitating illness, herbal tonics will help to strengthen the vitality of the lungs and the system in general. These should be continued for several months: Gentian, Mullein, Lungwort, Chamomile, Burdock and Elecampane.

Poisoning

1. IMMEDIATE TREATMENT IS ESSENTIAL FOR ALL POISONS.
2. DO NOT INDUCE VOMITING.

   If lips or mouth show signs of burning: Cool by giving water or milk to drink.

   If unconscious or convulsing: Place gently on side with head sideways in recovery position to clear airways and prevent choking. Do not give fluids. Do not induce vomiting.

   If breathing or heartbeat have stopped: Begin resuscitation immediately. Take care not to contaminate yourself with poison that may be round the child's mouth.
3. IF SERIOUS RING AN AMBULANCE.

   Collect samples of vomit and containers such as bottles, etc.

   If you know what poison your child took, see below.
4. NOTE: Poisoning must be treated seriously. Please refer to specific chapters in this book to treat the remaining symptoms once medical treatment has been given.

HOW TO USE: HERBS, PAGE 16 | HOMOEOPATHICS, PAGE 20 | CELL SALTS, PAGE 25

Psoriasis

An acute or chronic inflammatory skin disease often inherited.
Metabolic disturbances are common, specifically in the small
intestines where fat is improperly metabolized.

DESCRIPTION

A thick layer of whitish or silvery scales, usually on knees, elbows,
scalp and trunk. May also be on nails, palms and soles. Itching is
mild, if any. There may be reddened areas of skin. Scratching causes
bleeding but there is no flow of fluid such as occurs in eczema.

WHAT TO DO

- Avoid refined, processed foods, soap, sugar and sugar products,
  fatty foods, eggs, dairy products, citrus fruit and citrus juice
- Expose skin to sunshine, seawater or salt baths once weekly; or
  $^1/_2$ cup cider vinegar in bath water to restore acidity
- 2–3 drops of Lavender Oil can be added to bath water
- Wash hair with Jojoba Shampoo and rinse with $^1/_2$ cup cider
  vinegar to 1 litre ($1^3/_4$ pints) water
- Good foods to eat: carrot, beetroot, cucumber, grape, sesame
  seed and sesame oil.

Herbs
Internally: To purify the blood, stimulate the liver and help metabolic processes, combine any of the following and drink regularly for three weeks, stop for one week, then repeat: Burdock,
  Dandelion, Sassafras, Red Clover, Slippery Elm and Valerian.
External application: Marshmallow or Comfrey Ointment can be
  helpful.

Homoeopathic
We advise that you seek the help of an experienced natural health
practitioner, the following remedies are a guideline only. Natural
remedies can offer significant help to sufferers of psoriasis.

Arsen Alb 6c: Thickened skin which burns, itches and swells.

Graphites 6c: Eruptions worse behind ears, palms or backs of hands, bends of joints and folds of skin.

Kali Brom 6c: A leading remedy especially if child is the nervous type, and no clear symptoms arise.

Lycopodium 6c: Dry, withered, scaly eruptions.

Petroleum 6c: Rough, cracked and leathery; itchy, worse on hands and in cold weather.

Sulphur 6c: Dry, scaly, unhealthy skin; heat and itching of scalp which is dry and worse from washing.

Cell Salts

Calc Fluor: For thick, tough, cracked skin.

Calc Phos: For red, itchy skin.

Kali Phos: For nervous child.

Kali Sulph: For peeling skin.

These can be combined favourably and taken daily for at least three weeks, stop for one week, and repeat if necessary.

HOW TO USE: HERBS, PAGE 16 | HOMOEOPATHICS, PAGE 20 | CELL SALTS, PAGE 25

Rheumatic Fever

Believed to be a long-term complication from Streptococcus A-type infections. Inflammation of the connective tissue in joints, heart and blood vessels.

Complications: Bronchopneumonia, pleurisy, chorea (involuntary flicking movements), skin eruptions, heart disorders such as change in normal rhythm of heart beats, heart murmurs (due to heart valve damage), galloping heart tones, heart failure.

DESCRIPTION

May be sudden onset of pain and stiffness in one or more joints; often moving to other joints; sweating; fever; rapid heart beats; appetite loss. May be slow onset with fatigue, general ill health and weight loss. May be increased number of white blood cells.

WHAT TO DO

SEEK MEDICAL ADVICE

Because of complications, place child under the care of experts in the medical and natural health field. (A throat culture is essential.)

Bed rest, calm and a stress-free environment are needed. Give a liquid diet initially – plenty of fluid – apple juice or apple cider vinegar/water.

Later add citrus fruits, greens and root vegetables, fish and white meats.

Avoid: Meat, egg, dairy products, pickles, refined carbohydrates, sugar and spices, rhubarb, gooseberries, coffee and tea.

Massage: Helps stimulate circulation to the affected parts and prevents toxic deposits from settling in joints.

Herbs

To help remove stress and calm the heart especially: Skullcap, Passionflower, Hawthorn, Valerian, Mistletoe or Motherwort.

To induce sweating and lower fever: Yarrow, Elder, Peppermint or Pleurisy Root.

To stimulate appetite and remove fatigue: Ginger, Gentian.

For pain: Lobelia.

External application: Lavender, Peppermint or/and Rosemary Oils can be rubbed onto the skin at site of painful joints. Mix 2–3 drops with 2–3 tsp Soya or Almond Oil and massage.

Lobelia and Hypericum Tinctures can also be rubbed onto affected parts.

Homoeopathic

Aconite 30c: Restless and thirsty with fever and dry, hot skin. Scanty urine, stitching pain in chest, hot, pale or red swelling of joints, restless and shifting from one place to another.

Belladonna 30c: High fever, joint pains come and go suddenly.

Bryonia 30c: Intense fever, frontal or back headache, acute stitching pains, rapid, violent heartbeat, sour sweat worse from slightest motion even of breath.

Calc Carb 30c: Brought on maybe by working in water. Heat and sweat of head; cold, clammy feet and hands; violent perspirations about 3 a.m. Pain is worse from movement.

Rhus Tox 30c: Relief from continued motion; worse damp weather, cold and approaching storm. Tearing pains with paralyzed sensation and stitches. (Follows Bryonia well.)

Streptococcin 30c: For complications or lack of recuperation.

(Other useful remedies: Arnica, Colchicum, Dulcamara, Pulsatilla, Sulphur, Spigelia.)

Cell Salts

Ferr Phos: For first stage of fever, congestion and pain; rapid, throbbing pulse.

Alternate Ferr Phos with Kali Mur: When above fever signs occur with inflamed joints and swelling. Thumping pulse heard all over body. Thickening of tissues during fever.

Calc Phos: Weight loss, debility, run-down and exhausted.

Alternate Calc Phos with Nat Phos: When fever comes on very slowly.

Nat Phos: Sour-smelling sweat; creamy yellow tongue; acid taste in mouth.

HOW TO USE: HERBS, PAGE 16 | HOMOEOPATHICS, PAGE 20 | CELL SALTS, PAGE 25

Ringworm

Caused by a fungus often transferred from a young animal.

DESCRIPTION

Small, circular patches of raised skin – rose-coloured and scaly. The centres heal, leaving red rings. On the scalp it appears as small, round, bald patches. Usually appears first on head (in hair), then on chest, back of abdomen and often the groin. However, any area can become affected.

It is contagious on contact.

WHAT TO DO

- Wash the infected part every day with soap and water. Use separate towels, flannels, etc.
- Keep the area dry and exposed to air or sunlight
- Change clothing (especially socks) frequently and whenever sweaty
- Check animals to prevent cross-infection.

Herbs

Blood purifier for ringworm: Poke Root.

Antiseptic: Golden Seal. Use as a tea and also to rinse the infected scalp.

External: Clean and dry affected skin with Thuja Tincture. Oil of Lavender, Teatree or Thyme can be applied together or separately (2 drops of each to 3 tsp Olive or Soya Oil).

Homoeopathic

Sepia 6c: For isolated ringworm-type spots. May be itching, redness and rawness.

Rubella

An infectious disease.

Rubella (German Measles) is an acute, infectious disease, milder but sometimes difficult to distinguish from measles (see also Scarlet Fever).

DESCRIPTION

Begins as a mild headache and fever (37.5–38°C/99.5–101°F), stiff neck, slightly runny nose and dry throat. The glands are often swollen behind the ears.

A rash appears on the face and neck on the first day, then moves to the trunk and limbs. There may be fine, pink spots around the mouth and some pinkness of the eyes though not weeping.

The rash and fever seldom last more than five days. Rubella is more severe in females.

Most common season: spring or early summer.

Incubation period: 2–3 weeks.

Isolation period: Until rash fades.

Recovery time: 2–5 days.

WHAT TO DO

Herbs

To relieve pain: Jamaica Dogwood or Hops.

To help relax: Elder or Chamomile.

For fever: Catnip, Yarrow, Boneset or Lemon Balm

To provide extra nourishment during illness: Lavender, Thyme or Juniper.

Combine your choice of herbs and have child sip warm throughout the day. Sweeten with honey if desired.

Homoeopathic

After suspected contact, see Resistance and Immunity, page 29.

HOW TO USE: HERBS, PAGE 16 | HOMOEOPATHICS, PAGE 20 | CELL SALTS, PAGE 25

Rubella 30c (Nosode – see page 31): To help clear a severe case or for lingering after-effects of the disease. *Do not give whilst disease is incubating.*

For other useful remedies, see Measles.

Cell Salts

Ferr Phos: Gradual onset, fever, rosy spots on cheeks, chilly with sweats, wants head cool.

Kali Mur: For coated tongue, swollen glands and runny nose. Alternate with Ferr Phos if these symptoms exist.

PLEASE NOTE

There is great danger of foetal deformity if pregnant women are exposed to Rubella, especially during the first trimester.

SEEK MEDICAL ADVICE OR HOMOEOPATHIC ASSISTANCE.

TO BUILD RESISTANCE

To help strengthen the immune system and restore to full health after the disease (or vaccination), see page 29.

Scabies

A skin infection by an animal called an itch mite.

The female is just visible to the naked eye; yellowish-white with eight legs. She burrows into the skin and lays her eggs, then dies. The eggs hatch in six days and leave the burrow in larval form, growing quickly to adults so the disease may be fully developed in two weeks. Frequently, the burrows are not visible.

Spread by close bodily contact with an infected person and through infected bedding, etc.

Scratching can cause severe inflammation or secondary infection such as impetigo (school sores).

DESCRIPTION

Intense itching, especially when child is warm. The burrow in the skin is distinctive and seen as a greyish or white hair-like line, often zigzag, about 0.5–1 cm (about $1/4$ in) along the skin with a dark speck at the farthest end (the eggs). Usually found in webs and sides of fingers, backs of hands, lower abdomen, penis and lower buttocks, underarms, elbows and on palms and soles of feet in younger children.

WHAT TO DO

Daily washing of body and clothes is essential.
Keep clothes and bedding separate to prevent possible spreading.
Lemon and Garlic juice mixed together makes a useful application
    to affected parts.

Herbs
Internal: Cleansers may help make conditions unpleasant in the skin layers and help drive the mites out. Elecampane Root, Fumitory, Figwort and Aniseed mixed can be drunk as a tea daily.

HOW TO USE: HERBS, PAGE 16 | HOMOEOPATHICS, PAGE 20 | CELL SALTS, PAGE 25

External application: Oils of Clove, Lavender, Thyme and/or Peppermint (1–2 drops) mixed with Soya or Almond Oil are rubbed into affected parts several times daily.

Tansy Tincture or Infusion can be added to bath water or used to bathe body.

Homoeopathic

Arsen Alb 6c: Eruption on bends of knees: pustular eruptions with burning and itching, worse from external warmth.

Lycopodium 6c: Violent itching causing thickening of skin; worse from warmth of bed and hot applications; better when uncovered.

Mercurius 6c: Itching which is worse in bends of elbows; large, pustular eruptions.

Sulphur 6c: Tingling and itching with burning and soreness after scratching.

Psorinum 30c: Once only for repeated outbreaks of single, pustular spots after main eruption has gone.

(Others: Nux Vomica, Hepar Sulph, Causticum.)

Cell Salts

Calc Sulph taken internally 3–4 times daily; can also be crushed and applied locally to the affected parts.

Note: Hydrocortisone creams may be effective in the short term but can worsen the condition in the long run.

Scarlet Fever

An infectious disease.
An acute disease caused by a streptococcal bacteria producing a fever, sore throat and characteristic rash.

DESCRIPTION

Begins abruptly with headache, vomiting, fiery-looking throat with gradually increasing severity. The tongue is furry and throat and palate become bright red.

On the second day, the child has a bright, deeply-flushed face ('scarlet face'), except an oval white area around their bright red lips. The rash is flushed skin with minute points of intense red which usually starts on the neck and spreads over the body and limbs. It does not occur on the palms of hands and soles of feet. After about a week, the rash fades from the neck and peeling begins and may continue for several weeks.

Most common season: winter (and maybe autumn).

Incubation period: 1–7 days.

Isolation period: For seven days from the date of onset of the disease and until all symptoms have subsided, all abnormal discharges have ceased, and all open lesions have healed.

Recovery time: About three weeks.

Complications: Rheumatic fever, nephritis, ear infection, sinusitis, pneumonia.

SEEK IMMEDIATE MEDICAL ADVICE

Symptoms of swollen neck glands, earache, dark-red or smoky urine, swelling around eyes or painful joints can indicate complications such as Rheumatic Fever, Nephritis, Ear Infection, Sinusitis, Pneumonia.

The following procedures can be helpful in restoring to full health *after medical treatment* or *until medical aid arrives*.

HOW TO USE: HERBS, PAGE 16 | HOMOEOPATHICS, PAGE 20 | CELL SALTS, PAGE 25

WHAT TO DO

Restricted diet during high fever: fresh fruit, vegetables, soups and freshly squeezed fruit or vegetable juices, or water. By taking no proteins, the body can use its energy to fight off the infection instead of digesting unnecessary food.

Herbs

To soothe: Slippery Elm or Marshmallow.
To cleanse: Golden Seal, Dock, Mullein and/or Red Clover.
To provide extra nourishment: Lavender, Juniper and/or Thyme.

Homoeopathic

After suspected contact, *see* Resistance and Immunity, page 29.

Apis 30c: High fever, no thirst, prickly skin, scanty urine; child is drowsy, restless and agitated.

Belladonna 30c: Sore throat, strawberry tongue, swollen glands; rash is smooth and bright red. Delirium.

Bryonia 30c: For very slow appearance of rash; or sudden disappearance of rash with onset of complications.

Chamomilla 30c: If throat becomes ulcerated and child has a suffocative cough.

Rhus Tox 30c: Child is drowsy, weak, depressed and restless; tongue is red and smooth, eruption does not appear.

Sulphur 30c: If rash is rough and dark-coloured.

Scarletinum 30c (Nosode – see page 31): To help clear a severe case or for lingering after-effects of the disease. *Do not give whilst disease is incubating.*

Cell Salts

Ferr Phos: High temperature, headache, sore throat.
Kali Mur and Kali Sulph: Alternate every two hours after Ferr Phos.
Calc Phos: For convalescence period.
Kali Phos: If exhaustion is extreme, with putrid sore throat – give half-hourly until improvement.

TO BUILD RESISTANCE

To strengthen the immune system and help restore to full health after the disease, see page 29.

Shock

A condition caused by a lack of blood supply resulting in a lowering of the activities of the vital functions. It may be the result of illness, injury, bleeding, burns, repeated vomiting, diarrhoea, severe pain, heart failure or allergic reactions (e.g. to bee stings).

DESCRIPTION

- Skin is pale, cold and clammy, with profuse sweating
- May feel faint or giddy or have blurred vision
- May feel sick and vomit
- May be thirsty
- May be anxious
- Pulse tends to increase in rate but weaken as shock deepens
- Breathing is shallow and rapid.

WHAT TO DO

1. *Seek expert help.*
2. Lay patient down in Recovery Position with head lower than rest of the body and turned to the side if possible with one leg tucked up (unless unconscious, vomiting or if injuries make this inappropriate).
3. Reassure and give Aconite 30c.
4. Loosen clothing at the neck, chest and waist.
5. If thirsty, moisten lips with water.
6. Protect with blanket or sheet where needed.
7. Keep record of pulse and breathing rates.

Homoeopathic
Aconite 30c: Shock with great fearfulness and anxiety.
Arnica 30c: If as the result of any injury.
Carbo Veg 30c: Extreme cases, semi-conscious; cold breath and body; pale or blue.
Coca 30c: Altitude sickness, confusion, double-vision.
Ignatia 30c: Emotional shock.
Veratrum Album 30c: Restless, chilly, profuse cold sweat, watery diarrhoea.

Sinusitis

An inflammatory condition of the sinuses occurring during common colds and nasal catarrh.

DESCRIPTION

Starts as a heavy feeling in the face and head, especially when bending forward. First, a copious discharge from the nose. Next, the nasal passages swell and mucous or pus collect in the sinus cavities behind the nose and cause great distress. The resultant pressure causes severe tenderness, pain and headache, sometimes toothache. Whereas a cold should clear up in a few days, untreated sinusitis can last for weeks.

WHAT TO DO

Exercise, good ventilation, nourishing diet. Avoid mucous-forming foods, especially dairy foods.

Drainage points on the face can provide relief when massaged. Massage drainage points by applying on/off pressure (3-second intervals) down sides of nose, along cheek bones, around bony orbits of eyes and temples as often as needed for relief.

Herbs

If eyes are affected: Eyebright

To help dry out tissues and remove catarrh: Golden Seal, Bayberry, Elder, Golden Rod, Yarrow.

To soothe inflamed surfaces: Marshmallow.

As antiseptic and to help fight infection: Echinacea, Garlic.

To clear overloaded lymphatic system: Poke Root.

Inhalation: Peppermint, Eucalyptus and/or Teatree Oils (4 drops) can be added to a bowl of steaming water and breathed in while holding towel over head to retain steam.

External application: Rub above-mentioned oils on painful parts (1 drop of each to 2 tbsp Soya or Almond Oil).

Homoeopathic

Hepar Sulph 30c: Pain in facial bones; boring pain in upper lids worse from dry, cold winds and draughts. Red, inflamed eyes and lids; sore nostrils with thick discharge.

Iodum 30c: Sneezing; dry nose, fluent and hot in the open air; helps relieve a copious discharge; pain in eyes; throbbing head as of tight band; pain at root of nose and frontal sinuses; loss of smell.

Kali Bich 30c: Pressure and pain at root of nose. Thick, greenish-yellow discharge or bright yellow. Sore nasal bones; tough elastic plugs leaving raw surface. Violent sneezing. Profuse, watery or stopped up sensation. Headache over eyebrows with aching and fullness worse over left eye.

Kali Iod 30c: Violent headache; pain through sides of head over eyes and root of nose; red, swollen nose. Profuse, hot, watery discharge. Sneezing, stuffy or dry with no discharge.

Phosphorus 30c: Over-sensitive smell; chronic catarrh; tired eyes worse from light; fullness in head.

Cell Salts

Ferr Phos: Fever and congestion; pain in sinuses; flushed face; rapid pulse; throbbing pain.

Kali Mur: Dull pain in sinus; thick, white discharge; stuffed-up head.

Nat Mur: Nasal obstruction, loss of smell; sensation of beating hammers in nose, worse from cold air.

Kali Sulph: Yellow, slimy discharge, worse in warm room and evening.

Silica: Chronic thick, offensive, acrid discharge; ulceration of mucous membranes; chronic nasal catarrh.

SEEK HOMOEOPATHIC OR MEDICAL ADVICE

If condition fails to respond in a week.

HOW TO USE: HERBS, PAGE 16 | HOMOEOPATHICS, PAGE 20 | CELL SALTS, PAGE 25

Sleep

1 Insomnia

Children who are happy and active during the day are probably having enough sleep. Children have differing sleep requirements, some children needing a lot less sleep than others the same age and size.

Sleep provides rest for the brain and nervous system.

Insomnia is caused by a functional disturbance of the brain – the blood-flow to the brain doesn't slow down as it should at bedtime.

Possible causes: Putting children to bed before they are tired; physical discomfort; excess noise; extreme temperatures; hunger; digestive disturbances; fear; worry; overexcitement (e.g. after stimulating games or television programmes); inability to relax.

WHAT TO DO

Prolonged use of sedatives may be harmful and addictive.

A warm bath with 2–3 drops of Lavender Oil or Valerian tea added to bath water.

Cool bath and brisk skin rub in the morning.

Adequate ventilation in the bedroom.

A light evening meal (preferably no more than two hours before bedtime).

If child has no allergy problems, a hot milk drink can be relaxing.

Adequate exercise during the day but not overstimulation as overtiredness can also contribute to insomnia.

Reading a bedtime story initiates a 'slowing down' process and gives the child quality time with the parent.

Herbs

To help calm the nervous system: The following Calcium-rich herbs Valerian, Hops, Catnip, Chamomile and/or Passionflower may be taken in the evening before bedtime.

Homoeopathic

Aconite 30c: Restless sleep, tossing and turning, worse from fear or fright.

Arsen Alb 30c: Very anxious and restless, cannot stand to lie in bed, worse after midnight.

Coffea 30c: Cannot rest the mind, worse from excitement. Acute senses, hears distant noises distinctly.

Ignatia 30c: Worse from grief, e.g. during parent's absence.

Nux Vomica 30c: Cross and tired in the morning. May waken with headache. Sleepy in the early evening but wakens 3–4 a.m.

Passiflora 30c: General insomnia remedy. Useful if the other remedy pictures don't seem to fit.

Pulsatilla 30c: Wide awake in the early evening before midnight.

Sulphur 30c: Catnaps; slightest noise awakens, then going back to sleep is very difficult.

Cell Salts

Ferr Phos: Drowsy in the daytime, but sleepless at night.

Kali Phos: For children who cry and scream during sleep; dream; twitch muscles; yawn; stretch or sleep walk. Give with warm drink before bed and again in bed if necessary.

Nat Phos: Insomnia associated with stomach pain or discomfort.

Silica: For nervous excitable children who feel the cold.

2 Nightmares

- Child may wake crying or screaming from a bad dream
- Child may scream, toss and turn, sit up and talk, but doesn't wake up or remember in the morning
- Sleep walking.

HOW TO USE: HERBS, PAGE 16 | HOMOEOPATHICS, PAGE 20 | CELL SALTS, PAGE 25

Some causes: Excessive or unwise eating before bed; fever; fear of the dark; family stresses.

WHAT TO DO

Herbs
Take Vitamin B and C-rich herbs such as Mistletoe, Chamomile, Thyme, Valerian, Hops or Skullcap (especially for sleepwalking).

Homoeopathic
Calc Carb 30c: Horrid visions on opening eyes; jerks and jumps at noises; sleep talking, night sweats; confused and frightened on awakening.

Helleborus 30c: Uneasy sleep with dark floating visions; sudden screams but cannot be fully aroused.

Lycopodium 30c: Many frightful, anxious, vivid dreams, of murder and accidents.

Phosphorus 30c: Constant dreams, irrational talking; starts up suddenly when falling asleep; anxious upon awakening.

Pulsatilla 30c: Jerking limbs, confused dreams; suddenly sitting up in sleep; maybe screaming during sleep.

Stramonium 30c: Half-slumber; intense fear of the dark and of shining objects; awakens terrified; dreams and visions when half asleep.

Cell Salts
Calc Phos: Vivid dreams – dreams of fire and danger.

Kali Phos: Useful for sleepwalkers; highly-strung nervous children.

Nat Sulph: Heavy sleep with anxious and plentiful dreams.

Bach Flowers may also be useful to work on emotional aspects (books on Bach Flowers and the Bach Flower Remedies can be found in most health shops.)

Spots and Rashes

This section gives possible causes for spots and rashes.
Refer to individual headings elsewhere in the book for what to do.

Allergy
If none of the other possibilities prove to be the cause, or if rash appears only at certain seasons or after exposure to certain foods or otherwise, suspect an allergy. See Allergy (page 39).

Bites
Usually obvious, as there are only a few in isolated areas.

Chicken Pox
Small, raised, irritating spots that turn to watery blisters and form crusts. Usually start on the trunk, then the limbs and face. Can turn septic.

Contact Dermatitis
May appear as any one of a range of pimples or rashes, and cause mild or severe irritation. Caused by sensitivity to a specific substance. To determine this, see Contact Dermatitis (page 194).

Eczema
Itchy, red skin which may weep a clear fluid after scratching; forms crusts when dry. Skin becomes less red, dry and thickened. Starts in bends in knees and elbows in toddlers; cheek and foreheads in babies.

Hives
Very itchy red spots of varying sizes; may cover large parts of the body; they become swollen and elevated then disappear and reappear.

Impetigo
Red spots progress to watery blisters then pus-filled sores which discharge and spread the infection. This leaves raw skin which

HOW TO USE: HERBS, PAGE 16 | HOMOEOPATHICS, PAGE 20 | CELL SALTS, PAGE 25

eventually forms crusts. Usually starts around mouth and nose or in armpit and groin in babies.

Measles
Rash of red-pink blotches beginning on face or behind ears, maybe in the mouth and spreading to trunk and limbs. Accompanied by 'cold' symptoms. High temperature; sore runny eyes irritated by sunlight. Rash becomes raised and blotchy.

Nappy Rash
Scalded skin on bottom and nappy area.

Psoriasis
Thick layer of silvery scales, mild itching if any; scratching easily causes bleeding; usually on knees, elbows, scalp and trunk.

Ringworm
A circular patch of raised, rose-coloured, scaly skin. The centre heals to form red, scaly rings. In the hair it leaves bald patches. Usually starts on head in hair, chest, back and abdomen.

Rubella
Similar to measles, but with a milder illness; spots are smaller and a paler pink. Just before the rash appears, lymph nodes behind and below back of skull swell.

Scabies
Itchy skin often without rash, worse in the groin and underarm. Generally doesn't affect the head or neck. Distinguished by the burrow seen as a grey or white hairlike line along the skin about 0.5–1 cm ($1/4$ in) long with a darker speck at the farthest end although in most cases the burrow is not visible.

Scarlet Fever
Small bright red spots that are close together, usually start on neck, back and chest; accompanied by headache and vomiting, sore throat, high temperature; flushed skin but pallid around mouth.

Sprains and Strains

Sprain: Stretching or tearing of a ligament.
Strain: Overstretching of a muscle or tendon.
Causes: Both can be caused by sudden wrenching or twisting of any joint.

DESCRIPTION

Pain, loss of power, tenderness. Worse when attempting to move the limb. With sprains there is marked swelling and discoloration due to bleeding beneath the surface. Fractures can occur with sprains (see page 109).

WHAT TO DO

- If there is any external bleeding, deal with this first (see Wounds).
- Avoid massage.

Apply the 'RICE' Formula (the first five minutes is important):

Rest: Ensure that injured limb is completely rested.
Ice: Make an ice pack by crushing ice into towel or plastic bag, or by simply using a pack of frozen vegetables (oil can be put onto skin first, for sensitive skin). You *must* have something between the ice and skin, or you risk an ice burn. Repeat ice packs for no more than ten minutes in every hour, for first 24 hours.
Compression: Apply a tubigrip around injury. If the limb becomes painful, cold or numb, or the tubigrip feels too tight, remove it. Any rings on fingers should be removed, and the bandaging should be removed at night.
Elevation: Keep the limb raised as much as possible.

The healing process is greatly aided by stimulating the blood flow and relaxing the tense muscles.

After resting the injured limb for 24 hours, continue the RICE treatment combined with *gentle* exercise. Take the limb through the normal range of movement, stop if pain is excessive, apply ice imme-

HOW TO USE: HERBS, PAGE 16 | HOMOEOPATHICS, PAGE 20 | CELL SALTS, PAGE 25

diately after exercise. Do not force movement of the injured limb.

Note: Achilles rupture should have immediate assessment by a medical practitioner. Ligaments that are completely torn are often not painful, but are of greater significance as the joint is unstable.

Herbs
To help reduce swelling and repair damaged tissue: Apply a *poultice* of Chickweed, Comfrey or Puriri.
If skin is not broken: Arnica Ointment several times daily.
If skin is broken: Calendula Cream or Lotion several times daily.
For pain: Oils of Wintergreen, Sage, Rosemary or Thyme (5 drops mixed with 3 tsps Olive or Soya Oil) can be rubbed gently on to painful part. Avoid rubbing oil into deep cuts.

Homoeopathic
Arnica 30c: For sudden wrenching of muscles with injuries to the soft tissues of the body. Half-hourly for 3-4 doses, followed by Rhus Tox 30c twice daily for 4-5 days.
Bryonia 30c: If any movement hurts, but also seek medical advice. After a few doses go back to Rhus Tox to help repair injury.
Ledum 30c: If affected parts feel numb or cold and feel better after cold applications. Then resume taking Rhus Tox to help repair injury.
Rhus Tox 30c: For injuries to ligaments and fibrous tissues.
Ruta Grav 30c: For old sprains causing lingering problems.

Cell Salts
For Sprains:
Ferr Phos: Sprains, muscle pain, worse from movement.
Kali Mur: Sprains with bruising and swelling.
These can be used internally and as a lotion to bathe the affected part (four crushed tablets mixed with $1/2$ cup of water).
For Strains:
Alternate Kali Mur and Calc Fluor for no more than two weeks.

> **SEEK MEDICAL ADVICE**
> If there is no improvement after two days using above procedures.

Teeth

1 Teething

There are a number of ways you can help your baby through the stressful and often painful periods of cutting teeth.

Herbs
Catnip or Chamomile tea is a safe and soothing drink for babies. This may be sweetened with honey if desired. A few drops of Plantago Tincture may be added to this drink, or rubbed onto the painful gum area to ease pain. Rub 1 drop of Clove Oil onto gums.

Homoeopathic
Calc Carb 30c: Difficult teething with lots of saliva and easy bleeding and swelling of gums, diarrhoea. Stools sour with undigested food.

Calc Phos 30c: For slow teethers who are weak and tired during the teething stage. Foul hot spluttery stools may be watery. Teeth decay rapidly. These children are often slow in learning to walk.

Chamomilla 30c: One cheek may be red, hot or swollen; child cries and is very dissatisfied; convulsions may accompany teething. Yellow-green slimy stools smelling like bad eggs. Pain is intolerable. Head and scalp are hot and sweaty.

Kreosotum 30c: Teeth decay rapidly; child worries and frets, must be patted all night.

Cell Salts
Calc Phos: For slow cutting teeth; also for rapidly decaying teeth, or deformed teeth especially when accompanied by runny stools.

Calc Fluor: Vomiting and crying during teething. Lack of enamel.

Nat Mur: Constant dribbling of saliva during teething.

HOW TO USE: HERBS, PAGE 16 | HOMOEOPATHICS, PAGE 20 | CELL SALTS, PAGE 25

2 Toothache

Usually caused by decay. Take good care of first teeth. If they decay, then the second teeth will also be troublesome.

Toothache may also be caused by taking food or drink too hot or too cold, or exposure to cold air.

A decayed tooth must always be dealt with by a dentist or dental nurse.

WHAT TO DO

Foods to ensure healthy teeth in the long term: almonds, apples, carrots, celery, cheese, buttermilk, nuts, oats, rye, radish, sunflower seeds, alfalfa (lucerne).

Herbs
Combine your choice from the following lists:

To ensure healthy teeth in the long term: Comfrey, Sage, Myrrh, Plantain and/or Yarrow.

To relieve acute pain: Lobelia, Clove or Plantago Tinctures – 1–2 drops on cotton wool and applied directly to painful tooth.

For unhealthy, ulcerated, easy-bleeding gums, poor teeth and bad breath: Echinacea, Myrrh or Poke Root.

Homoeopathic
Aconite 30c: For throbbing, burning pain.

Belladonna 30c: Throbbing gum, dry mouth, ulcerated gums.

Coffea 30c: For unbearable pain, worse from heat, better from cold drink.

Kreosotum 30c: Early decay of teeth; teeth turn yellow then dark.

Mercurius 30c: Aching teeth, worse at night with bad breath, moist mouth, easy bleeding and swelling of gums, inflamed or abscessed roots, increased salivation and sensation as if the teeth were too long or too loose.

Plantago 30c: Sensitive to touch, worse from cold air, better whilst eating.

Silica 30c: Deep pain and ulceration of gums. Abscesses about roots of teeth.

Cell Salts

Calc Phos: Useful after toothache to help purify blood throughout gums.

Calc Sulph: For abscessed gums which will not heal.

Kali Mur: Toothache with swollen gum or cheek.

Mag Phos: Nervous child with spasmodic, sharp, shooting pains. Better from hot applications.

Nat Mur: Toothache with excess saliva or tears, and easy bleeding gums.

Silica: Deep-seated pain and ulcerated gums.

Pressure Point: Apply firm pressure to index finger on the lower corner of fingernail nearest the thumb; may be necessary to apply pressure to both hands.

HOW TO USE: HERBS, PAGE 16 | HOMOEOPATHICS, PAGE 20 | CELL SALTS, PAGE 25

Throat (Sore)

May be the beginning of a cold or the first symptom of a more serious illness. Watch for changes in symptoms and check under Cold, Scarlet Fever, Tonsillitis.

WHAT TO DO

Gargle with 2 tsp salt in 1 cup water: *do not swallow*.
Gargle with 2 tsp cider vinegar in 1 cup water.
Drink hot lemon juice and honey.

Herbs

To soothe a sore throat: Hyssop, Coltsfoot or Liquorice.
To purify: Elecampane.
To provide a natural source of vitamins and minerals: Sage and/or Thyme.

These herbs work well when mixed, drunk hot, sweetened with honey.

Inhalation: Oils of Lemon, Sage and/or Thyme (2 drops of each) added to a bowl of steaming water. Cover head with towel and breathe in the steam to loosen the congestion and ease the pain.

Homoeopathic

Baryta Carb 12c: Can be taken night and morning for three days, then once weekly during susceptible time of year to help prevent recurrent sore throats with constantly enlarged tonsils.
Belladonna 30c: For throat that is sore, dry, red and inflamed.
Causticum 30c: Raw and sore throat.
Hepar Sulph 30c: Sticking pain as of a splinter in throat.
Mercurius 30c: Red, swollen, painful and very inflamed, with pains extending often to ears.
Rhus Tox 30c: Sore throat with swollen glands.
Streptococcin 30c: If throat has not been right since previous infection. Give once daily for two days.

Tuberculinum 30c: Recurrent sore throat spreading to chest with rattling wheeze. Give once daily for two days.

SEEK MEDICAL ATTENTION

If sore throat is very severe or if it doesn't improve within 48 hours.

HOW TO USE: HERBS, PAGE 16 | HOMOEOPATHICS, PAGE 20 | CELL SALTS, PAGE 25

Thrush

A fungal infection of the mucous membranes of the mouth in babies of both sexes or of vaginal tract in girls. The fungus is known as Candida Albicans.

DESCRIPTION

In mouth, thrush looks like milk curds but these will not brush off and may bleed when rubbed. These white patches occur on tongue, gums or throat. It may follow treatment by antibiotics. In vaginal infection, there is increased vaginal discharge and itching irritation outside the vagina.

WHAT TO DO

- Hygiene is important. For vaginal thrush, wash daily using herbal douche below and change underwear regularly. Care should be taken in using a douche on a young girl.
- Natural yoghurt can be very soothing when applied locally, but will not clear an established infection. Acidophyllus powder (break open a capsule) can be mixed with yoghurt prior to application for better results.
- Calendula or hypericum creams can be soothing when applied locally.

Herbs

Herbs can be used as a mouth wash, drink and/or douche:

Antiseptic: Golden Seal and/or Echinacea.
To soothe irritation: Raspberry
Douche: Add Cider Vinegar (1 tbsp per half litre/17 fl oz of water or above herb liquid) to help maintain correct pH level.
To rinse mouth or vaginal area: Oils of Lemon, Geranium or Sage (5 drops to $1/2$ cup water).

Homoeopathic

Candida Albicans 30c: Four times daily for two or three days.

Other useful remedies:

Arsen Alb 30c: Child thirsty for small amounts of water; great burning of affected parts.

Bryonia 30c: Nursing aggravates the sore mouth in babies.

Calc Carb 30c: For vaginal itching and whitish discharge.

Mercurius 30c: Gums are spongy, swollen and the sores tend to ulcerate. Diarrhoea may occur simultaneously.

Hypercal Lotion: Can be diluted (5 drops to $1/2$ cup water) to rinse mouth or vaginal area.

Cell Salts

Kali Mur: Will help soothe the itch. Suck tablets and use as wash (crush 4 tablets to $1/2$ cup water).

SEEK MEDICAL ADVICE

- For stubborn recurring cases.
- There are advanced balancing techniques now available which enable the body to repel the invasion of Candida Albicans. Your nearest Touch For Health instructor should be able to help or advise you.

HOW TO USE: HERBS, PAGE 16 | HOMOEOPATHICS, PAGE 20 | CELL SALTS, PAGE 25

Tonsillitis

A specific infection of the tonsillar tissues (these are two small lumps visible on each side of the throat near the base of the tongue) and associated glands.

Usually a streptococcal infection that some children cannot easily fight off. See also Throat (Sore) page 176.

DESCRIPTION

Acute Tonsillitis: Fever, loss of appetite, coated tongue, difficulty swallowing, maybe headache and vomiting.

When pushing down on the tongue with a spoon handle, the side walls of the throat appear red, swollen, possibly with whitish-yellow spots.

In younger children there may also be abdominal pains.

Chronic Tonsillitis: Less severe than acute condition but more persistent. General ill health, easily tired, poor appetite, repeated sore throats, low-grade fever and enlarged neck glands.

Adenoids often enlarge with chronic tonsillitis, which can cause blockage of air through the nose. This results in mouth-breathing, producing a nasal voice and snoring.

Repeated ear infections are more common.

WHAT TO DO

> ### SEEK MEDICAL ADVICE
>
> For chronic Tonsillitis, we advise that you seek the help of an experienced natural health practitioner.

Give child mainly liquid foods such as fresh, unsweetened juices and soups, plus fresh fruit and vegetables until acute symptoms subside.

Best foods are carrot, celery, beetroot, pineapple, lemon and coconut milk.

Hot lemon and honey drinks.

Cider Vinegar gargle to break up mucous (1 tsp per $^1/_2$ cup water).

Cool compress to throat at night, if throat feels hot, or child
desires it.

Herbs

Antiseptics, blood purifiers and soothing herbs are best suited. In
chronic cases, continue for three weeks, stop one week and repeat
again.

Make a mixture of any of the following blood-purifying herbs:
Golden Seal, Burdock, Echinacea, Poke Root, Queens Delight
(especially if ears are involved).

To help soothe inflamed surfaces: Marshmallow, Liquorice and/or
Slippery Elm.

To provide extra nourishment: Rosemary, Cloves and/or Teatree.

Homoeopathic

Arsen Alb 30c: Burning, swollen throat better from warmth; worse
from cold and swallowing.

Baryta Carb 30c: Constantly enlarged tonsils. Also glands of neck
and behind ear are swollen. Helps remove a predisposition to
tonsillitis.

Belladonna 30c: Dry and angry-looking but inclined to swallow
often. Sharp pains in tonsils.

Hepar Sulph 30c: Sensation of splinter in throat, or sharp, throbbing
pains with formation of pus.

Lachesis 30c: Bluish-red swelling, worse from anything tight
around throat, worse from hot drinks or swallowing, and worse
in the morning.

Mercurius 30c: Raw, burning, maybe yellow spots, stitching feeling
towards ear on swallowing. Enlarged tonsils may cause difficulty in breathing.

Rhus Tox 30c: For chronic tendency to sore throat with loss of
appetite.

HOW TO USE: HERBS, PAGE 16 | HOMOEOPATHICS, PAGE 20 | CELL SALTS, PAGE 25

Cell Salts

Ferr Phos: For first signs of throat problem, take internally and use as a gargle (4 tablets crushed and mixed with $1/2$ cup water).

Calc Phos: If swelling has continued for a long time.

Calc Sulph: If pus forms.

Kali Mur: Swollen tonsils, painful swallowing, white tongue.

Nat Phos: Yellow coating at base of tongue, with feeling of lump in throat.

SEEK MEDICAL ADVICE

For developing earache or rash, marked swelling of neck glands, swollen joints, dark red or smoky urine passed in small amounts.

Travel Sickness

The rhythmic or irregular movement associated with travelling affects the balance mechanism of the inner ear and, via the nerves, disturbs the digestive system, causing nausea and vomiting.

WHAT TO DO

- Plenty of fresh air in the vehicle.
- Keep mind busy and stretch legs to keep up circulation; reading tends to make the problem worse.
- Have child exert on/off pressure firmly at the following places:
  Find the little dent on the skull about half an inch back from the ear;
  Also press with fingertips firmly into the middle of the tummy just below the rib cage.
- Special strips available from chemists give relief when placed on wrists. These work on the principle of Acupuncture.

Herbs

Have child sip tea made from Clove, Peppermint, Basil and Cinnamon half an hour before travelling. Combine or use separately, and place 3–4 drops on handkerchief to sniff during the journey: Clove, Peppermint, Basil and Cinnamon Oils.

Homoeopathic

Give the remedy you choose, once the night before and once on the morning of the journey; also once when the journey begins. If the journey is long, you may need to repeat the dose at half-hourly intervals.

Belladonna 30c: Air sickness or earache from pressure during flying.

Borax 30c: Worse from downward motion in cars or planes.

Cocculus 30c: Worse from food smells and watching motion; nausea with faintness, vomiting and trembling; better lying down. This is a particularly useful remedy.

HOW TO USE: HERBS, PAGE 16 | HOMOEOPATHICS, PAGE 20 | CELL SALTS, PAGE 25

Ipecac 30c: Heavy vomiting associated with travel sickness.

Petroleum 30c: Empty feeling, nausea with empty stomach; worse from fumes, light, noise and sitting up. Particularly useful.

Tabacum 30c: Seasickness, icy, cold sweat; nausea; terrible, faint, sick feeling at pit of stomach; worse having eyes open and better from fresh air. Particularly useful.

Cell Salts

Nat Phos and Kali Phos together at half-hourly intervals. Give these half an hour before leaving also.

Urinary Tract Infection (Cystitis)

The urinary tract can cope with a few germs but if the body defences are down and excess germs build up in the urethra an infection can get underway. As the infection spreads, the bladder loses its ability to hold increasing amounts of urine without discomfort. Urination becomes painful and is followed by painful spasms. Infection can eventually travel to kidney, causing back pain, elevated temperature, sweating, shivering, headaches and general ill feeling.

WHAT TO DO

- *Drink a little water often.*
- Acidify the urine by drinking 2 tsp apple cider vinegar with 1 tsp natural honey in a glass of water with each meal.
- Keep genital area clean, especially in girls; wash well; wipe from front to back after bowel movements *not* back to front.

Herbs
It is advisable to continue taking the herbs for several weeks.

For infection: Uva Ursi and Buchu.
To soothe the irritated area: Marshmallow.
To help cleanse and ease the passage of urine: Lavender and/or Juniper.
Chronic Cystitis: When the above herbs fail to be of any use, change to regular drinks of Echinacea, Burdock, Golden Seal and Myrrh. These act as a natural antibiotic.
External application: Oils of Lavender or Juniper (2 drops) can be mixed with 3 tsp Olive or Soya Oil and rubbed on to the lower abdomen often.

Homoeopathic
Aconite 30c: Burning, cutting, scanty urine with agony beforehand.
Belladonna 30c: Cramps in bladder with frequent, profuse, dark urine. Sensation of something moving inside.

HOW TO USE: HERBS, PAGE 16 | HOMOEOPATHICS, PAGE 20 | CELL SALTS, PAGE 25

Berberis 30c: If the pains have moved to the back or hips as well as the bladder region. Sticking tearing pain worse from deep pressure. Cutting pain in bladder with burning on urinating. Back feels stiff and numb.

Cantharis 30c: Violent inflammation with intolerable urging. May be blood in the urine. Urine is passed in drops, with intense burning on urinating. Aching in small of back.

Staphysagria 30c: For cystitis resulting from sexual activity.

Tuberculinum 30c: Chronically recurring cystitis, when above remedies fail. Then go back to the indicated remedy if infection recurs.

Cell Salts

Kali Phos: Itching, scalding, bloody urine, cutting pain.

Mag Phos: Painful straining, severe spasms.

Nat Mur: Frequent with burning, cutting pain.

SEEK MEDICAL ADVICE

For recurrent infections, your local medical doctor will take a urine culture before advising. You can get asymptomatic bacteria in the urine, which may cause renal damage so ensure that a medical practitioner follows up a cystitis symptom. Especially in boys as they will require investigation of the renal tract. A homoeopath may also be able to help remove the cause of the problem. Vaginal discharge associated with sexual activity must always be checked by your doctor.

Warts

A common viral disease of the skin. Left untreated, warts may spontaneously remit because the body develops an immunity to the wart virus. Few warts are contagious.

WHAT TO DO

Vitamin E capsules can be squeezed on and covered with a plaster. Repeat continuously for 2–3 weeks.
Aloe Vera can be applied the same way.

Herbs
Greater Celandine leaves can be picked and the yellow sap squeezed on to the wart daily until wart goes.
Thuja Tincture can be painted directly on to warts.
The juice of the Milkweed can be applied directly to warts daily.
Lemon Oil can be dabbed on before bed every night.

Homoeopathic
Causticum 6c: Small warts all over the body, especially nose, fingertips, eyebrows.
Ferr Pic 6c: Warts cover the hands.
Nat Mur 6c: For warts on the palms.
Nitric Acid 6c: Large, jagged, easy-bleeding warts.
Thuja 6c: A general wart treatment. Warts can be large and painful.

Cell Salts
Kali Mur and Silica: 1 tablet of each three times daily.

Note: 'Magic' cures are many, varied and at times successful, and should not be discounted.

HOW TO USE: HERBS, PAGE 16 | HOMOEOPATHICS, PAGE 20 | CELL SALTS, PAGE 25

Whooping Cough

An infectious disease.
An acute, infectious disease affecting the air passages with characteristic coughing spasms.

DESCRIPTION

Appearing in stages: First stage lasts from 3–7 days and consists of a runny nose, sneezing, slight fever, and cough which is worse at night, comes in spasms, and becomes progressively stronger.

During the second week (stage 2) the coughs are so close together that the child cannot draw another breath and appears to be suffocating.

The air is then sucked in which such force that it produces the characteristic whoop. After several such spasms (lasting 2–3 minutes) the child perspires, brings up some thick, slimy mucous and may vomit food. This leaves the child exhausted and frightened but he/she recovers and can be quite happy between attacks. There may be 40–50 attacks daily.

Young infants and immunized children who develop whooping cough may have all the symptoms *without* the whoop.

Most common season: spring and autumn. Age: under five.

Incubation period: 7–14 days.

Isolation period: For three weeks from the date of onset of the typical spasms.

Recovery time: Mild cases with no whoop: 7–10 days. More serious cases can last from three weeks to two months.

Complications: Include brain damage, pneumonia, convulsions and dehydration.

WHAT TO DO

- Give fluids – fresh fruit and vegetable juices, broths. Overloading the stomach with food is to be avoided; also avoid cold draughts.
- Keep warm and well rested. Be prepared for vomiting.
- Reassure child during spasms; *support – do not suffocate.*

Herbs

Make a mixture from the following:

To purify glands: Red Clover or Thyme,
To soothe respiratory passages: Mullein or Marshmallow.
To calm the child: Chamomile or Lavender.
To tonify the system: Gentian.

Homoeopathic

After suspected contact, see Resistance and Immunity, page 29.

Antim Tart 30c: Worse from drinking and eating, cries before cough, vomits large amounts of mucous; nausea and cold sweat, white-coated tongue.

Belladonna 30c: Stomach pain and tears before spasms, dry throat, coughs until mucous comes up, excited by tickling in throat.

Bryonia 30c: Must sit up to cough. Coughing and vomiting occurs during a meal; yet child can return easily to finish the meal.

Carbo Veg 30c: When child is absolutely worn out, pale and exhausted from the disease.

Cuprum 30c: For convulsions following a coughing spasm.

Drosera 30c: Barking cough so frequent that child chokes; raising of phlegm ends in retching and vomiting, worse after midnight.

Ipecac 30c: Stiff and blue during spasms, with difficult breathing; nausea better from vomiting; copious discharge and perspiration; exhausted after attack.

Cell Salts

Calc Phos: Weak constitution or lingering cases.

Kali Mur: Alternate with Mag Phos where there is thick, white mucous.

Mag Phos: For first sign of illness.

HOW TO USE: HERBS, PAGE 16 | HOMOEOPATHICS, PAGE 20 | CELL SALTS, PAGE 25

SEEK MEDICAL ADVICE

Child has convulsions; shortness of breath *between* spasms, or the child becomes debilitated during the long illness.

TO BUILD RESISTANCE

To strengthen the immune system and restore to full health after the disease or vaccination, see page 29.

Worms

The most common worms are threadworms (6–9 mm/$^1/_4$–$^1/_3$ in long). These look like fine cotton threads. Eggs are laid on the outside of the anus and are transferred from there back to the mouth or to toys, etc.

DESCRIPTION

Itching around the anus, which may disturb the child's sleep. Child may grind teeth in sleep. Sometimes the worms move into the vagina, causing itching and discharge.

Examination of the stool will usually show fine moving threads; worms can often be seen around the anus whilst child is sleeping. Symptoms are general irritability, usually large appetite with low corresponding weight gain; child bores fingers into nose; there may be dark rings under eyes.

WHAT TO DO

- Ensure the child washes hands with soap after going to the toilet.
- Keep fingernails short.
- Prevent the child from scratching; wear gloves if necessary.

Herbs

Choose: Wormwood, Tansy and/or Southernwood and mix with Chamomile to improve the taste. Mix with honey if necessary and have child drink this 2–3 times daily until symptoms are clear.

Further helpful herbs to be added and continued daily: Peppermint, Thyme or Garlic.

Raisins soaked in Senna tea may be an easy food for the young child.

HOW TO USE: HERBS, PAGE 16 | HOMOEOPATHICS, PAGE 20 | CELL SALTS, PAGE 25

Homoeopathic

Abrotanum 30c: Pale and old-looking face with blue rings around eyes; child is cross and peevish; ravenous hunger but no weight-gain.

Absinthium 30c: Grinding teeth, loathing of food with uncomfortable, irritable feeling in stomach, and colic in abdomen.

Calc Carb 30c: Swollen abdomen; dark rings under deep-seated eyes; sore nostrils; ravenous hunger.

Cina 30c: Rings around eyes, grinds teeth; picks and rubs nose; night terrors; hungry soon after eating; itchy anus.

Cell Salts

Kali Mur: Alternate with Nat Phos when child has an itching anus and white tongue.

Nat Phos: For round, long or thread worms, combined with squinting and twitching of facial muscles.

Give 1 tablet twice daily between meals. Stop and if no improvement after five days combine Nat Mur and Silica and take in the same dosage.

Wounds

1 Superficial (cuts and abrasions)
2 Deep (lacerations, incisions, punctures, contusions – internal haemorrhage).

1 Superficial wounds

Where only the upper layers of the skin are damaged or removed; some bleeding occurs but mostly a clear fluid exudes. This may be from graze, or a slight cut with a sharp instrument.

- Clean using Hypercal Lotion (10 drops to $^1/_2$ glass water) as antiseptic and healer, and follow if necessary with Calendula Cream and plaster.

2 Deep wounds

Lacerations: Full thickness of skin is cut through often in an irregular fashion. Caused by a jagged or blunt instrument – infection is common. The edges can be pulled apart. There may be damage to the underlying tissues (muscles, nerves, blood vessels); these are often pulped and contain dirt.

Incised wounds: Skin is cut by a sharp instrument so that skin is divided and there may be damage to deeper tissues such as nerves, tendons or blood vessels.

Punctures: Skin is pierced by a sharp point such as a nail or rose thorn. There is damage to deep tissue and, as oxygen cannot get to the injured part, infection often results. This type of wound is particularly prone to the tetanus bacteria.

Contused wounds: Internal haemorrhage – damage to the soft tissue beneath the skin. Caused by a knock from a blunt object. May be a cut but the more serious damage is beneath the skin, with pain, swelling, bruising and thickening of tissues.

HOW TO USE: HERBS, PAGE 16 | HOMOEOPATHICS, PAGE 20 | CELL SALTS, PAGE 25

GENERAL PROCEDURE FOR ALL DEEP WOUNDS

1 Seek medical advice
Give Arnica 30c for shock and bleeding. Follow advice given in a regular First Aid book, such as St John Ambulance.

2 Control bleeding
- *Elevate the part* with cut surface uppermost.
- *If blood is spurting*, it is from an artery – ensure there is nothing sharp in the wound, then apply pressure around wound.
- *If blood is from a vein* only light pressure is necessary.
- *If you suspect a fracture or if a bone or sharp object is poking through*, apply pressure alongside object or bone, place pads of cotton wool or soft material round the wound to a height to prevent pressure on object or bone; bandage diagonally so as to slow bleeding but not press on object. Bleeding can be stopped by applying pressure at an appropriate point between heart and wound. Do not apply pressure for more than fifteen minutes.
- *For contused wounds*, elevate the part and apply ice packs (or ice in plastic bag) and a firm bandage.

3 Clean the wound when bleeding has stopped, with cotton wool soaked in one of the following:

- Hypercal Lotion (5 drops in $^1/_2$ glass water)
- Comfrey Lotion (see Herbs page 16).
- Teatree Oil (3 drops to $^1/_2$ cup water).

Gently stroke foreign matter out, using a clean cotton ball for each stroke.

Note: Do not use Arnica on an open wound. If child's cuts tend to go septic, place a few drops of Urtica Urens or Hypercal Lotion in the daily bath water.

Compress or ointment
To soothe the wound: Marshmallow, Comfrey or Slippery Elm.
To disinfect and prevent infection: Golden Seal, Elecampane, Sage or Lavender.
To help heal: Calendula, Comfrey.

4 Bandaging
Soak a piece of gauze or lint in lotion made from your chosen herbs. Cover entire wound. Repeat with a second piece of gauze (this can be replaced later without disturbing the dressing immediately next to the skin). Bandage firmly or use butterfly plasters (these can be home-made easily by cutting plaster into butterfly shape).

5 If wound becomes inflamed, i.e. red and hot with swelling and tenderness, or starts discharging, remove outer gauze and replace with clean gauze soaked in Hypercal Lotion or above-mentioned herbs. Re-bandage. Give Homoeopathic Hepar Sulph 30c three times daily until discharge stops. However, if no improvement after two or three days, treat as for Infection.

6 When wound begins to heal it can gradually be exposed to the air, as oxygen plays an important part in the healing process.

INTERNAL APPROACH TO HELP HEAL WOUNDS

Herbs
Comfrey, Elecampane, Golden Seal and Rosemary can be taken as a tea to help fight infection from within.

Homoeopathic
Lacerations: Often require skilled surgical treatment.
Arnica 30c: For shock and to help control bleeding.
Hypericum 30c: If pain is severe.

Incised Wounds:
Staphysagria 30c: For very deep painful wounds.

Punctured Wounds:
Ledum 30c: To help guard against any tetanus bacteria. Four times daily for two days.
Hypericum 30c: Use instead of Ledum especially for shooting pains in the wound. This will also help guard against tetanus bacteria.

HOW TO USE: HERBS, PAGE 16 | HOMOEOPATHICS, PAGE 20 | CELL SALTS, PAGE 25

Contused Wounds/Internal Haemorrhage:
Arnica 30c three times in one day followed by Arnica 30c for the
next few days to allay pain and promote absorption of blood.
Give Ledum 30c if parts feel numb and cold, it feels better with cold
application and if there is delay in appearance of the bruise.
Veratrum Album 30c: Internal bruising where swelling and pain
occurs.

Blows to Chest: Bryonia 30c

Blows to Head: Nat Sulph 30c

Blows to Abdomen: Veratrum Album 30c

Cell Salts
Calc Sulph: For those wounds which are filled with pus.
Ferr Phos: For first stage of cuts, bruises, falls and sprains.
Kali Mur: Give for swellings.
Alternate Kali Phos and Nat Phos for signs of infection (e.g. redness
and swelling).
Silica: For neglected wounds that are slow to heal, or infected.

SEEK MEDICAL ADVICE

- If you suspect damage to deeper structures, or internal
  haemorrhage. Symptoms of this will be: pain, tenderness,
  cold clammy skin; restlessness; thirst; or dizziness and
  fainting.
- If despite above procedures, there is increased pulse; paleness; distressed breathing or a deteriorating condition.
- If foreign body is embedded – this may be large or small
  (e.g. pieces of glass).

Miscellaneous Ailments

BAD BREATH
This can be seen as an early warning sign and may indicate: liver trouble, inadequate digestion of food, tooth decay, respiratory problems, gum infection, inflammation of the throat, catarrhal discharge or sinus trouble.

It is wise to seek advice from a natural health practitioner at this early stage to help isolate the cause.

CONTACT DERMATITIS
Inflammation of the skin, arising from touching a substance to which the person is sensitive. The eruption appears within a few minutes to hours after contact or application, developing rapidly and vanishing some variable time after removal of the cause.

Description:
The eruption may be spotty, discoloured, raised or flat, bleeding or pus-filled, pimples, blisters or cuts.

Sensations present upon the skin may be: itching, pricking, tingling, smarting, burning, painful. Variations in intensity of these sensations depend upon susceptibility and sensitivity of the individual.

What to do:
A patch test with suspected substances will usually cause a reaction within 20 minutes (place on soft skin like wrist). Seek advice from a Touch For Health instructor (muscle testing will isolate suspect substances which then need to be eliminated or rebalanced).

Homoeopathy offers antidotes to the offending substances to counteract ill-effects. And, even if the cause is eliminated, homoeopathic remedies are often helpful in restoring the skin to normal by treating the whole constitution.

Herbal lotion to give relief in the meantime:
3 tsp either of cold pressed Soya, Almond or Castor Oil mixed with
    1 drop each of Oil of Lavender and Geranium.
Chamomile and Hyssop extracts are also soothing.

HOW TO USE: HERBS, PAGE 16 | HOMOEOPATHICS, PAGE 20 | CELL SALTS, PAGE 25

GROWING PAINS

Any unexplained, vague, temporary bone pains that the child complains of, providing such pains do not follow an acute illness (e.g. Rheumatic Fever) or an injury (e.g. broken bones), are usually called 'growing pains' and can often be helped by:

Daily drinks of Parsley Tea which is rich in vitamins and minerals;
Calc Phos Cell Salt taken three times daily;
Homoeopathic Phosphoric Acid, Guiacum or Calc Phos 30c or Belladonna 30c.
A few drops of Lavender or Thyme Oil can be rubbed onto the affected area to soothe.
Seek medical or homoeopathic advice if pains persist.

HEAD LICE

A form of louse (Pediculosis Capitis) that lives exclusively on the scalp. The adult lice are light green in colour, visible to the naked eye and live at the base of the hair. They lay their white eggs onto the hair shaft and reproduce rapidly. They spread mostly through personal contact or by the use of infested head garments, combs, pillows etc.

Description:
The white, glistening nit or egg can be found glued firmly and in great numbers to the hair shaft, especially around the ears and in mid-back of head. Severe itching of scalp. Constant and vigorous scratching causes oozing of a fluid that is watery at first but in severe cases contains blood or pus. The fluid dries and forms crusts or may remain sticky and mat the hair.

What to do:
A medical shampoo can be obtained from pharmacies to kill the nits.
During treatment, keep bedding, brushes, combs, etc. clean and separate to avoid cross-infection.

Herbs:
Apply Aniseed Oil to the infested areas to kill nits and eggs; or mix one part Sassafras Tincture with two parts Olive Oil and rub over scalp before shampooing, four times weekly. Comb with a fine-

tooth comb to remove dead lice and eggs. Repeat daily until hair is cleared and lice and eggs are gone.

Seek homoeopathic advice if the scalp has been badly affected. Useful remedies are Oleander, Vinca Minor, Viola Tric and Pediculosis Capitis.

HYPERACTIVITY

A condition where the child is unable to relax, rest, sleep or concentrate to the same extent as others of a similar age. Hyperactivity is nearly always the manifestation of an allergy. The most common allergens are sugar, wheat products, dairy products, corn, eggs and nuts. A child can have a mild or severe allergy to one or several foods at the same time. For what to do, see Allergy, page 39.

HYPERVENTILATION

Abnormally rapid breathing which has the effect of reducing the carbon dioxide content of the blood, causing the brain cells to receive less oxygen. This leads to dizziness and even unconsciousness and a lowering of the blood pressure.

Hyperventilation may occur in altitude adjustment; some respiratory diseases such as bronchial asthma; anxiety; or for no obvious reason.

Attend to the cause.

PENIS INFECTION

Signs of this are swelling, inflammation, pain and redness which is worse from urinating. It can be caused by foreign matter collecting under the foreskin and is usually more common where the foreskin is overtight; it can also be caused by a urine infection.

Herbs:
Golden Seal herb can be taken internally 4-5 times daily for a few days until inflammation subsides.

Homoeopathic:
Aconite 30c: Give at first sign for crawling, stinging pain which comes on suddenly. Urine is red, hot and painful or difficult to pass.

HOW TO USE: HERBS, PAGE 16 | HOMOEOPATHICS, PAGE 20 | CELL SALTS, PAGE 25

Cantharis 30c: Raw, burning pain with intolerable urging to urinate. Urine is scalding.

Merc Corr 30c: Penis and testicles are enormously swollen, red, sore and hot with intense burning on urinating. Use in conjunction with medical advice.

Externally: For local redness use Hypercal Lotion to cleanse and disinfect.

SEEK MEDICAL ADVICE

Immediately.

SMELLY FEET

Most common causes of smelly feet are: undesirable bacteria or fungi; or emotional problems (worry, fear or anxiety can cause profuse sweating of the feet)

Bathe feet: To water, add a few drops of Pine Oil or Witch Hazel Tincture to bathe the feet.

If emotional, there are books on Bach Flowers available in most health shops; or seek advice from a natural health practitioner skilled in emotional work or a One Brain or Touch for Health instructor.

SWOLLEN TESTICLE (Hydrocele)

This is an accumulation of clear, watery, light yellow-coloured fluid in the sac around the testicle. It may develop at any age. In babies it usually resolves without medication. In older children swelling of a testicle could be serious and needs a medical diagnosis. Therefore, **seek medical attention** in all cases. It is caused by some mild irritation in the lining of the sac. It may occur on both sides but more often only on one. The tendency is for a gradual size increase. There is little or no pain, and it does not seem to affect the general health or be annoying, unless the sac grows to a considerable size. Once medical attention is sought, the condition may be helped by daily drinks of Golden Seal and Parsley. Common homoeopathic remedies useful for this condition are Apis, Conium, Graphites, Iodum,

Fluoric Acid or Pulsatilla. The choice will be dependent upon the total symptom picture – see Remedy Pictures – or seek advice from a homoeopath.

Cell Salts required for this condition are Calc Fluor and Kali Mur, which can be alternated daily.

Note: Swelling of testicle may also be due to Mumps (page 138).

UNDESCENDED TESTICLES

About two months before birth, the testes descend into the scrotum (the skin-covered bag suspended from the groin). Occasionally, one or both testicles fail to descend. If both, this may lead to sterility in the adult. A good place to check is when the boy is in a warm bath, as the scrotum is relaxed. In cold weather the testes rise to the top of the scrotum.

Medically, this condition is corrected by hormone therapy or surgery if it does not resolve. (The concern is of developing cancer later in life in a testicle that cannot be checked.)

Homoeopathically, Thyroidinum 30c can be effective especially if the child's development in learning, speech or physical growth is slow.

The condition can also be approached from an emotional perspective, especially with the use of Bach Flower essences. The essences and books about them are available in most health shops. Seek advice from a natural health practitioner skilled in emotional work.

HOW TO USE: HERBS, PAGE 16 | HOMOEOPATHICS, PAGE 20 | CELL SALTS, PAGE 25

Remedy Pictures – Homoeopathic

ACONITE

General Characteristics: Mental and physical tension; healthy, strong types who suddenly come down with illness, haemorrhage, visual disturbances, fevers, restlessness, dry hot skin, great thirst and intolerance of warmth.

Sensations: Tearing, stabbing, cutting pains; numbness and tingling.

Modalities: Worse from exposure to cold, dry winds, draughts, frights, injuries, shocks, operations, evening, night. Better from fresh air.

ANTIMONIUM CRUDUM

General Characteristics: Great sadness, sulky, fretful, cannot bear to be touched or looked at. Gastric disorders worse from overeating. Thick milky white coating on tongue.

Sensations: Loathing of food; very tender feet when walking.

Modalities: Worse from extremes of heat and cold, cold bathing, heat of sun yet can also be better from heat.

ANTIMONIUM TARTUM

General Characteristics: Bad-tempered and complaining, worse from consolation and least touch; great drowsiness, cold sweats; great accumulation of mucous which is difficult to raise; pale, short of breath; heavily coated white tongue; desires but is worse from apples.

Sensations: Can't raise mucous, can't stand touch, shivering with cold then feverish heat.

Modalities: Worse from heat, cold, damp weather, evening and early night; anger or vexation.

APIS

General Characteristics: Anxiety with restlessness, great drowsiness; oedematous swellings; sleep disturbed by pain; anxious dreams with piercing screams during sleep; thirstlessness; complaints right-sided, or right to left.

Sensations: Burning, darting, stinging pains better from cold; sore sensitive skin worse from touch or pressure.

Modalities: Worse from all forms of heat; 4–6 pm; sleep.

Do not use before or after Rhus Tox.

ARNICA

General Characteristics: Great fear of being touched; over-sensitive to pain; injuries to soft parts; bruises, concussion; offensive discharges with odour of rotten eggs; helps prevent the formation of pus and blood poisoning.

Sensations: Bruised, sore feeling all over; bed feels too hard; head hot, body cold.

Modalities: Worse from rest and lying down. Better from motion.

ARSENICUM ALBUM

General Characteristics: Fastidious, sad and irritable; fear of death and darkness; great exhaustion yet restless, anxious and frightened especially during fever. Very chilly. Great thirst for small quantities at frequent intervals. Symptoms recur at regular time intervals.

Sensations: Burning pains better from heat; burning, scant discharges.

Modalities: Worse from cold, damp, midnight to 3 am, rest, lying with head low. Better from heat (except the head).

BELLADONNA

General Characteristics: Happy when well, violent symptoms, brain symptoms during illness can become wild delirium, illusions, moaning, jumping out of bed. Sudden local inflammations; fevers with flushed face, throbbing carotids; dry mucous membranes, sparkling eyes.

Sensations: Intolerable sensations, severe throbbing pain worse lying down, worse from heat. Chilly.

Modalities: Worse from cold, heat of sun, night, least jar, 3 pm to 3 am, right side. Better from warmth, resting, sitting up, lying on unaffected side.

BRYONIA

General Characteristics: Condition comes on gradually. Irritable. Useful for complaints coming on after suppressed discharges. Excessive dryness of all mucous membranes. Great thirst for large amounts. Constipation, gastric disorders with yellow-coated tongue; right-sided complaints. Lies very still, worse from least movement; worried and maybe delirious; wants to go home.

Sensations: Sharp, stitching pains, worse from motion, better from rest.

Modalities: Worse from slightest motion, at night about 9 pm or early am, heat of sun. Better from complete mental and physical rest, cool air and applications, lying on painful side.

Do not use before or after Calcarea Carbonica.

CALCAREA CARBONICA

General Characteristics: Slow mental and physical development; anxious, apprehensive; night terrors; slow to learn but tries very hard; difficult teething; easy sweat of head when sleeping; very chilly; sour smelling; enlarged glands.

Sensations: Craves indigestibles e.g. chalk, dirt, sand, has clammy legs, feet and hands.

Modalities: Worse from cold and damp, working in water, 2–3 am. Better from warmth but not overheating; when constipated; lying on painful side.

Do not use before or after Bryonia. Consult a homoeopath.

CARBO VEGETABILIS

General Characteristics: Lack of reaction to other remedies; extreme weakness after disease, especially due to loss of blood or other body fluids, haemorrhage; injuries; blueness with cold feet and legs, cold sweat, cold breath; very chilly with air hunger; excessive accumulation of gas worse upper abdomen, better from passing wind. All food disagrees; very offensive discharges.

Sensations: Burning or painful. Hoarseness and loss of voice worse in damp air and evenings.
Modalities: Worse from overheating. Better from being fanned.

CHAMOMILLA

General Characteristics: Teething problems. Nervous, excitable types who are intolerant and over-sensitive to the least pain. Spiteful, irritable, quiet only when carried, impossible to please. One cheek flushed and hot, the other pale and cold. Diarrhoea smelling of rotten-eggs, worse during teething.
Sensations: Local heat of hands and feet and one cheek; hot discharges e.g. stools and sweat.
Modalities: Worse from heat, evening, night, teething, sensitive to damp, cold and wind on ears.
Do not use before or after Nux Vomica.

CHINA

General Characteristics: Very regular recurrence of symptoms e.g. every second day. Great debility from discharges. Hypersensitive to criticism or touch. Anaemic. Excessive flatulence not relieved by belching. Very disturbed digestion.
Sensations: Tearing, drawing pains, bodily soreness worse from rest, better from mild movement. Painlessness of discharges; singing in ears; throbbing, bursting headaches.
Modalities: Worse from cold, damp, autumn, least touch, least draught of air, any mental or physical exertion. Better from warmth and hard pressure.

CINA

Pale-faced children who pick their nose, grind their teeth at night; white discoloration around mouth. Ravenous appetite, bad-tempered, dislikes cuddles. Worm infestations.

COCCULUS

General Characteristics: Cannot bear the least contradiction. Travel sickness with dizziness. Nervous temperaments. Colic not relieved by passing wind.
Sensations: Numbness, parts go to sleep, emptiness in organs, trembling and weakness, feeling of sharp stones in abdomen.

Modalities: Worse from travelling, loss of sleep, fresh air, mental and physical exertion.

DROSERA
Violent spasms, paroxysms of respiratory tract especially during acute illness like measles, whooping cough, etc. Can't get breath from coughing so much. Cough ends in choking, gagging, vomiting and cold sweat. Constant cough as soon as head touches the pillow. Coughs worse from lying down and after midnight; worse from warmth, drinking or using the voice.

EUPHRASIA
Profuse, bland discharges from nose with burning discharges from eye. Ailments from injuries especially to eye.
Modalities: Worse in evening or on rising in the morning, indoors, warmth, south wind. Better outdoors.

FERRUM PHOS
First stage of inflammatory processes e.g. fevers, haemorrhages etc. Worse 4–6 am and pm.

GELSEMIUM
General Characteristics: Lethargic, drowsy, dizzy, nervous, and hysterical. Physical complaints arising from nervousness e.g. diarrhoea before exams or new school. Dull headache with blurred vision and dizziness; first stage of fevers with aching back and limbs; chills and absence of thirst; watery discharges; influenza; loss of muscular coordination.
Modalities: Worse when left alone, warm moist weather, emotions, nerves, heat of sun and summer.

HEPAR SULPH
General Characteristics: When conditions show no sign of clearing up. Very chilly. Hypersensitive mentally and physically. Intolerant of pain, touch or draught of air. Sour-smelling excretions; profuse sweats. Use when pus has formed or is about to form; unhealthy skin, staphylococcal infections; injuries often become infected and are very sensitive to draughts or slightest touch. Croup worse from uncovering body parts.

Sensations: Sticking, throbbing pain. Sensation of splinter in throat. Very chilly.

Modalities: Worse from slightest draught, night. Better from mild, wet weather.

HYPERICUM

General Characteristics: Bad effects of head or spinal injury; pain after injuries or surgery; animal bites or scratches; helps prevent tetanus in puncture wounds.

Sensations: Excessively painful injuries to nerves especially fingers and toes; screaming from slightest motion of neck or arm; pains travel upward; during headache sensation of being lifted up high into the air.

Modalities: Worse from slightest motion of neck or arm; change of weather.

LEDUM

General Characteristics: Always cold, discontented and peevish. Alternating complaints, or symptoms appear diagonally opposite on the body. Helps prevent tetanus; punctured wounds, insect bites, rheumatic or arthritic complaints.

Sensations: Sticking, tearing, throbbing pain with no heat or swelling rapidly changing locality.

Modalities: Cold, yet worse from warmth of bed. Better from cool applications despite coldness.

LYCOPODIUM

General Characteristics: Intellectually keen types but physically weak, emaciated in upper parts of body. Fatigued, forgetful, lacks self-confidence, dislikes company but dreads solitude. Excessive flatulence, craves sweets; constipation predominates; urinary problems; dry skin, especially of palms; dryness of mucous membranes; nose full of crusts or plugs; twitching motion of nostrils.

Sensations: One foot hot the other cold. Right-sided complaints or right to left.

Modalities: Worse from both extremes of temperature but especially heat (except abdomen which is better from heat); exertion; 4–8 pm; sleep. Better from open air, uncovering, gentle motion.

MERCURIUS CORROSIVUS

Acute, violent inflammations e.g. of eyes, eyelids, kidneys, bowels. Dysentery, appendicitis, peritonitis.

MERCURIUS SOLUBILIS

General Characteristics: Changeable mental states: either slow to answer and despondent, or hurried, anxious and talkative. Dirty, yellow, rough complexion; violent toothache; weakness and trembling of all limbs; skin eruptions, ulcers or swollen glands, thin, burning, easy-bleeding discharges which can change to thick, yellow/green, bland discharges. Profuse sweat.

Sensations: Intense thirst despite moist tongue. Boring bone pains at night. Bad breath and bad taste in mouth.

Modalities: Worse from heat and cold, at every change especially to damp weather, all night; warmth of bed; lying on right side. Better from resting, high altitudes.

Do not use before or after Silica.

NATRUM MURIATICUM

General Characteristics: Anaemic, pale, greasy-looking complexions; emaciated about neck, old-looking children; depressed, emotionally sensitive to music; irritable at small noises; dry skin and mucous membranes or free watery discharges. Mapped tongue with dryness and thirst. Craves salt. Cannot urinate in the presence of others.

Sensations: Must have air but can get chilly.

Modalities: Worse from salt, seaside, company, consolation, heat especially close rooms, 9–11 am. Better from missing meals, being alone, loose clothing.

NATRUM SULPHURICUM

General Characteristics: Depressed, irritable when spoken to. Delirium. Mental as well as physical effects from blow to head. Saddened by music. Greenish-yellow catarrhs, diarrhoea on rising and moving about. Loose coughs better by sitting up and holding chest. Asthma.

Sensations: Can have violent, crushing, gnawing pain at base of brain.

Modalities: Worse from all forms of damp; sea air; daytime; lying on left side. Better in the open air.

NUX VOMICA

General Characteristics: Irritable, tense, impatient, spiteful, thinks everyone is against them; complaints from too much hard mental work, physically and mentally hypersensitive to pain, criticism, slight ailments. Stomach complaints from too much food causing retching and desire but inability to vomit. Drowsy in evening then wakeful 3–4 am. Reawakens at normal time feeling tired and worn out. Must be covered during fevers.

Sensations: Very chilly; great urging but difficult to vomit or pass stool.

Modalities: Worse from draughts, winter, open air, also dry weather. Better from warmth, rest, mild damp weather.

Do not use before or after Chamomilla or Zinc.

PHOSPHORUS

General Characteristics: Quick, lively, sensitive temperaments; rapidly growing, narrow-chested, stoop shouldered, indifferent, disinclined to mental and physical exertion. Slow, depressed yet can be excitable and enthusiastic in fits. Full of fears. Desires sympathy. Fidgety and restless.

Sensations: Burning in spots; intense heat running up back; emptiness. Fear strikes person in stomach. Hunger – must eat often. Craves salt and cold things. Great thirst but can vomit after drinking. Oppressed chest worse using voice, eating and drinking.

Modalities: Worse from cold (except stomach and head), thunder, weather changes, twilight to midnight, lying left side. Better from lying down and sleeping.

Do not use before or after Causticum.

PULSATILLA

General Characteristics: Gentle, yielding, unstable emotional temperament. Anaemic, pale-faced. Great changeableness of symptoms, shifting locality and sensation. Tearful, self-pity. Loves consolation. Can be submissive or obstinate, easily upset.

Changeable stools. Digestive complaints from overloading with rich, fatty foods. White-coated tongue. Sleepless early evening but sleeps late into morning. Copious greenish-yellow thick, bland discharges.

Sensations: Thirstlessness despite dry mouth. Chilliness despite being better in cool air.

Modalities: Worse from warm rooms, twilight to midnight, lying on left or painless side. Better from gentle motion in cool, open air despite feeling chilly.

PYROGENIUM

Septic blood conditions when other remedies fail to permanently improve. Horribly offensive excretions; tongue fiery red, clean and smooth. Very rapid pulse. Very restless and sore in bed. Complete inertia of bowel.

Sensations: Complains of bed being too hard; sweet but very foul taste in mouth.

RHUS TOXICENDRON

General Characteristics: Pains worse during rest and on beginning to move, yet better from continued motion; very restless during fevers with red, dry cracked tongue and triangular red tip. Sad, apprehensive, tearful worse at night. Acrid, foul secretions and excretions. Usually worse right side. Sprains and strains. Acute skin diseases. Conditions brought on by over-exertion.

Modalities: Worse from cold, wet weather, cold winds, getting wet especially after overheating, before storms, during and after rest. Better from warm applications; during warm weather.

Do not use before or after Apis.

RUTA GRAVEOLENS

General Characteristics: Mechanical injuries of bones; sprains, flat feet, overstrained eyes.

Sensations: Bruised pain, lameness; burning, aching, strained eyes.

Modalities: Worse from cold, wet weather, lying on painful part, outdoors, reading or straining eyes. Better from warmth and moving about indoors.

SEPIA

General Characteristics: Indifferent even to family. Melancholy worse from consolation and company. Tearful, disinclined to mental and physical labour. Hypersensitive to and irritated by noise and music. Constipation. Bed wetting. Easy sweating between folds of skin. Hair falls out.

Sensations: Chilly. Sinking feeling at 11 am not better by eating. Nausea at smell of food. Hates fats. Itching not better by scratching.

Modalities: Worse from stuffy rooms, before thunder, moist hot weather, excitement, milk. Better from violent exertion.

Do not use before or after Lachesis.

SILICA

General Characteristics: Lack of vital heat, icy coldness, light, fine types with dry skin, pale face, large sweaty hands. Nervous, anxious, timid but irritable if aroused. Melancholy, desires consolation. Lacks self-confidence yet gets through by sheer effort of will. Obstinate, headstrong, but cries with gentle treatment. Hypersensitive to noise. Slow learning to walk; weak ankles; sleep walkers. Longlasting suppurations, streptococcal infections; bad effects of vaccination; in-growing toenails; unhealthy, easily infected skin.

Sensations: Coldness from neck up over head to one eye, worse from draught and uncovering, better from wrapping up warmly. Stitching, stabbing, sticking pains worse from motion. Offensive foot sweat. Clammy hands and feet.

Modalities: Worse from cold, approach of winter, new and waxing moon. Better from warmth, wrapping head up warmly summer, humid weather.

Do not use before or after Mercurius.

SULPHUR

General Characteristics: Untidy, sedentary types, intolerant of bathing and covering, grumblers; variable hunger and thirst; can eat a lot and stay thin; likes sweets. Internal problems caused by suppressed skin eruptions. Relapsing conditions; lack of reaction to remedies in acute diseases. Skin eruptions worse from warmth and washing. Smelly eruptions and discharges.

Sensations: Scratching causes burning. Hands and feet burning hot in bed.

Modalities: Worse from heat, warmth of bed, standing still, bathing. Better from cold air.

THUJA

General Characteristics: Ailments from vaccination, especially diarrhoea. Depressed, dislikes company, quarrelsome, loss of memory, always hurried. Decayed roots of teeth. Greasy complexion, especially forehead. Unhealthy skin. Green, offensive, catarrhal discharges. Constipation or sudden, gurgling diarrhoea. Overgrowths of tissues, e.g. warts, moles, styes. Sweats only on uncovered parts or all over except head especially while sleeping. Deformed, brittle nails.

Sensations: Strange, fixed ideas (of something alive in abdomen; of soul and body being separated; of limbs being made of glass; of domination by a superior being).

Modalities: Worse from damp, cold air, bathing, heat of bed; am and throughout day or after 3 am and 3 pm. Better from scratching, stretching, after sweating.

Remedy Pictures – Cell Salts

CALC FLUOR
Found in surface of bones, tooth enamel and in elastic fibres of skin, muscular tissue and blood vessels. Deficiency causes relaxed tissues and elastic fibres, e.g. unnaturally loose teeth, varicose veins or haemorrhoids.

Modalities: Worse from damp. Better from rubbing and applications to affected parts.

CALC PHOS
Found in bones, teeth, connective tissue, blood and gastric juice. Deficiency causes slow teething, anaemia, bone diseases, poor digestion.

Modalities: Worse from cold, motion, getting wet, change of weather. Better from rest, warmth, lying down.

CALC SULPH
Found in skin, cells and blood. Deficiency causes slow healing of wounds, excessive formation of pus – catarrh, boils, ulcers, abscesses, pimples. Pus is thick, yellow and sometimes blood-streaked.

Modalities: Worse from getting wet, washing or working in water.

FERR PHOS
Found in blood. Deficiency causes fever, inflammation, poor appetite, weight loss. Tongue clean, red, inflamed or swollen.

Modalities: Worse from motion. Better from cold.

KALI MUR

Found in blood, nerve cells and muscles. Deficiency causes glandular swellings, liver troubles. Thick, white, sticky discharge. Tongue has white-grey coating. Ulcers, blisters on tongue.

Modalities: Worse from motion; rich, fatty foods.

KALI PHOS

Found especially in brain and nerves; also in muscle and blood. Deficiency causes irritability, fearfulness, exhaustion. Tongue brown or mustard-coloured, dry or inflamed; breath is offensive.

Modalities: Worse from noise, physical or mental exertion, cold air, beginning movement after rest. Better from gentle motion, eating, rest, excitement.

KALI SULPH

Carries oxygen to cells of skin and mucous membranes. Deficiency causes lack of oxygen in skin with resultant chilliness and desire for fresh air. Especially useful in later stages of inflammation where discharges are yellow, slimy, sticky or greenish. Tongue is yellow and slimy. Loss of taste.

Modalities: Worse from warm room; towards evening. Better from cool, fresh air.

MAG PHOS

Found in nerves and muscles. Deficiency causes cramps, spasms, convulsions, toothache, sharp shooting pains. Especially indicated in lean, thin people with highly nervous temperaments.

Modalities: Worse from touch, cold wind, washing. Better from application of heat, firm pressure, friction and bending double.

NAT MUR

Found in every liquid and solid part of the body. Acts upon the lymphatic system, blood, liver, spleen, mucous lining of alimentary canal. Deficiency causes fluid imbalance, e.g. bloated skin or excessively dry skin. Loss of taste or salty taste. Frothy saliva. Failure to respond to other cell salts.

Modalities: Worse from seaside, cold weather, morning.

NAT PHOS

Found in blood, muscles, nerve cells, brain cells and intercellular fluids. Deficiency causes excess acidity in system, worms, gastric disturbances from overfeeding on milk and sugar. Coppery or acidic taste in mouth. Sour-smelling discharge. Tongue thick, yellow moist coating.

Modalities: Worse afternoon or evening.

NAT SULPH

Found in intercellular fluid. Regulates quantity of water in body and eliminates excessive fluids. Deficiency causes swollen skin, liver diseases, bilious conditions. Tongue dirty greenish-yellow coating. Bitter taste in mouth.

Modalities: Worse from using water, living in low damp places, wet weather, eating watery plants, fish. Better from dry warm atmosphere.

SILICA

Found in blood, bile, skin, hair, nails, bones, nerves and glands. Deficiency causes slow formation of pus. Chilly sensitive people. Festering sores. Ulcers on tongue. Offensive thick yellow discharges.

Modalities: Worse from cold. Better from warm rooms, warm applications.

Bibliography

Airola, Paavo *How to Get Well* Health Plus Publications, Arizona 1974

Blackmore, M.C.H. *Mineral Deficiencies in Human Cells* Blackmore's Communications Service 1983

Boericke, *Materia Medica and Repertory* Jain Publications, New Delhi 1982

Borland, Douglas M. *Homoeopathy for Mother and Infant* British Homoeopathic Association, London

Chapman, J.B. *Dr Schuessler's Biochemistry* Thorsons Publishers Ltd, London 1973

Chatton, M.J., M.D. *Handbook of Medical Treatment* Jones Medical Publications 1977

Cox, Donavan & Heyne-Jones *Before the Doctor Comes* Thorsons Publications Ltd, London 1976

Fishbein, Morris, M.D. *The Handy Home Medical Adviser* Doubleday & Co, New York 1952

Gibson, Dr D.M. *Homoeopathy – First Aid in Accidents and Ailments* British Homoeopathy Association, London 1977

Green, Dr Christopher *Toddler Taming* Doubleday, Australia 1984

Houston, J.C., Joiner C.L. & Trounce, J.R. *A Short Textbook of Medicine* Hodder & Stoughton 1982

Kent, J.T. *Repertory of the Homoeopathic Materia Medica* Jain Publications, New Delhi 1985

Kichlu and Bose *Descriptive Medicine* Jain Publishing Co, New Delhi 1984 reprint

Lautié, Raymond, D.Sc & Passeberg, Andre M.D. *Aromatherapy* Thorsons Publishers Ltd, London 1979

Leavitt, Sheldon, M.D. *Homoeopathic Therapeutics as Applied to Obstetrics* A.P. Homoeopathic Library, Calcutta 1962

Lust, John *The Herb Book* Bantam Books, New York 1974

NZ Health Dept *Health & Development Record*

Palai Seul, Jean *Grandmother's Secrets* Penguin 1976

Pàlos, Stephan *The Chinese Art of Healing* Bantam 1972

Parker Merren *For Goodness Sake* Collins, Auckland 1978

Schuessler, Dr *Biochemic Pocket Guide* Pratap Medical
    Publishers, New Delhi

Shepherd, Dr Dorothy *Homoeopathy in Epidemic Diseases* Jain
    Publishing Co, New Delhi 1983 reprint

Speight, Leslie *Homoeopathy and Immunisation* Health Science
    Press, Essex, England 1983

Speight, Phyllis *Homoeopathic Remedies for Children* Health
    Science Press, Essex, England 1983

St Johns Ambulance *First Aid* Association & Brigade 1972

Woods, Dr H. Fergie *Homoeopathic Treatment in the Nursery*
    British Homoeopathy Association, London

Suppliers of Natural Remedies

(Country dialling codes: Australia (61); New Zealand (64); United Kingdom (44)). Natural remedies are easily obtained from health shops and some chemists. Their suppliers have mailing systems, so that you can order directly if you have difficulty obtaining remedies locally. Major suppliers in New Zealand, Australia and the United Kingdom are:

New Zealand homoeopathic suppliers:
Moores Pharmacy, Lincoln North Centre, 254 Lincoln Road,
    Henderson, Auckland. Tel: (09) 8368-576.
Selene Homoeopathics, P.O. Box 2456, Tauranga.
    Tel: (07) 5783-635.
Ushers Pharmacy (Naturopharm), 148–154 Tutanekai Street,
    Rotorua (P.O. Box 952). Tel: (073) 87-765.
Weleda NZ Ltd, P.O. Box 132, Havelock North.
    Tel: (070) 777-394.

New Zealand herbal suppliers:
Auckland Herbal Dispensary, 60 Waimarie Street, St Heliers.
    Tel/Fax (09) 5758-022.
The Herbal Dispensary, 220c Kilmore Street, Christchurch.
    Tel: (03) 3651-906.

Australian homoeopathic suppliers:
Brauer Biotherapics, 1 Para Road, Tanunda, South Australia.
    Tel: (08) 85 632-932
Martin & Pleasance, 26–30 Northumberland Street, Collingwood,
    Victoria 3066. Tel: (03) 9419-9733.
Newton's Pharmacy, 119 York Street, Sydney, N.S.W., 2000.
    Tel: (02) 9267 7889.

Australian herbal suppliers:
MediHerb Ptd Ltd, P.O. Box 713, Warwick, Queensland 4370.
  Tel: (07) 661-0700.
Pharmaceutical Plant Co., Unit 4, 385 Dorset Road, Boronia,
  Victoria 3155 or P.O. Box 68, Bayswater, Victoria 3126.
  Tel: (03) 9762-8677 or (03) 9762-8522.

United Kingdom homoeopathic suppliers:
Ainsworths, 40-44 High Street, Caterham, Surrey CR3 5UB.
  Tel: (01883) 340-332.
Helios, 97 Camden Road, Tunbridge, Wells, Kent N1 2QR
  Tel: (01892) 537-254.

United Kingdom herbal suppliers:
Baldwins (mail order amounts as small as 25 gms), 171–173
  Walworth Road, London SE17 1RW. Tel: (020) 7703-5550.
Hambledon Herbs (organic), Court Farm, Milverton, Somerset
  TA4 1NF. Tel: (01823) 401-205.
Herbal Apothecary, 103 The High Street, Syston, Leicester
  LE7 1GQ. Tel: (0116) 260-2690.
Neals Yard shops supply a wide range of herbs. These shops are
  now in many U.K. cities. Their central address is:
  Neals Yard, 3 Neals Yard, London WC2H 9DP.
  Tel: (020) 7379-1312.

Index

Page numbers indicated in bold should be looked up first.

128; watery 128–30; yellowy
125

Face, deeply flushed 158–9; pain
161–2
Faintness 113, 160
Fatigue, due to anaemia 42
Feet, smelly 197
Feeding problems, in babies 54; for
mothers 55–6
Fever **104–6**; & abdominal pain
128; bronchitis 63; & croup
87–8; fits 107–8; from
heatstroke 113–14; influenza
122–3; jaundice 124–7; measles
128–30; meningitis 131–3;
mumps 138–9; pneumonia
145–7; rheumatic fever 151–2;
tonsillitis 177–9
Fits 107–8
Flea bite 57–8
Foreign object, *see* Obstruction
Fractures 109–10; & bleeding 191

Gallstones 124–7
Giddiness 42; (*see also* Dizziness)
Glands, swollen, behind ears 154;
neck 159, 177–9; throat 177–9;
under jaw 174 (*see also* Neck,
stiff)
Glue ear 92–3
Groin, pain 196–7; swelling 197–8
(*see also* Testicles)
Growing pains 195

Haemorrhage, internal 190–3
Hay fever *see* Allergy
Head, bald patches in 153;
heaviness 161–2; lice 195–6
Headache **111 12**; & anxiety 45 7;
& eye strain 102–3; &
heatstroke 113–14; & hepatitis
115–17; meningitis 131–3;

scarlet fever 158–9; sinusitis
161–2
Health Kits, Cell Salts 26; Herbal
18; Homoeopathic 23
Hearing 93
Heat exhaustion 113–14
Heatstroke 113–14
Hepatitis 115–17
Herbs 16–19; forms: bath 19,
capsules 18, cleanser 30,
compress 19, cream 19, dried
17, fresh 17, inhalation 19,
lotion 19, oil 19, poultice
18–19, powders 17, syrup 17,
tablets 18, tincture 17, tonic 30;
& immunity 30; recommended
18; & resistance 30; use of,
external 18–19, internal 16–18,
in combination 27–8
Herpes simplex 77
Herpes zoster 71
HIV *see* AIDS
Hives 118–19
Homoeopathy, external use 23;
how much how often 22–4; how
to choose 21; how to take 22; &
immunity 31–2; in combination
21, 27–8; inimicals
(incompatible remedies) 21–2;
Miasms 24, 32; Nosodes 30–1,
in pneumonia 146;
recommended 23; Remedy
Pictures 199–209; & resistance
30–1
Hormones 134–6
Hydrocele (swollen testicle) 197–8
Hyperactivity 199
Hypersensitivity (Allergy) 39–41
Hyperventilation 45, **196**

Immune system **29–32**; &
immunization 31–2; Miasms 24,
32; & resistance 30–1

Nausea, & headache 111–12; & heatstroke 113–14; & travel 180–1
Navel, in babies 53–5; bleeding 55; oozing 55
Neck, stiff 131–3 (see also Glands)
Nightmare 164–5
Nipples, soreness in nursing mothers 55, 56
Nits, see Head Lice
Nose, bleeding 142–3; catarrh 138–9; congestion 141–2; discharge 75, 128–30, 141–2; & earache 93–6; inflammation 164–5; object in 143–4; runny 75, 128–30, 141–2
Nosodes, homoeopathic, & resistance 30–1; in pneumonia 147
Nursing mothers 55–6

Obstruction, in airways 73–4; of bile ducts 124; in ear 96–7; in eye 100; in lungs 73–4; in nose 143–4; in throat 73–4

Pain, abdominal 115–17; back 115–17; bone, over 109–10; chest 145–7; ear, in 93–6; ear, under 138–9; face 161–2; groin 196–7; growing pains 195; head 111–12; influenza 122–3; joints 151–2; kidneys 182–3; limbs 109–10, 122–3; lungs 63–5; muscles 168–9; penis 196–7; stomach 85–6; strains and sprains 168–9; & swelling after injury 109–10; teeth 170–2; when urinating 182–3
Pallor 42
Palpitation, due to anaemia 42; due to anxiety 45 (see also Pulse rate)

Penis infection 196–7
Periods, see Menstruation
Pneumonia 145–7
Poisoning 148
Poultice **18–19**, 33
Psoriasis 149–50
Pulse rate, decreased 125; rapid & weak 113, 160; no pulse beyond injury 109–10; to test for allergy 39–40
Puncture wounds 190
Pus, see Infection

Rashes 166–7; allergy 39; nappy 140
Remedy Pictures: cell salts 210–12, homoeopathic 199–209
Resistance 29–32; AIDS 37–8
Respiratory tract, infection 63–5, 77, 87–8
Rheumatic fever 151–2
Ringworm 153
Rubella 154–5

Scabies 156–7
Scalp, see Head
Scarlet fever 158–9
School sores 120–1
Sea sickness, see Travel sickness
Sepsis, see Infection
Shingles 71
Shock **160**; after birth 53–4, 55; in burns 67–70; electric 68; wounds 191
Sinusitis 161–2 (see also Congestion)
Skin (see also Spots & Rashes), abscess 33–4; allergy 39–41; in babies 54–5; bites 57–9, blisters 60; boils 61–2; bruises 66; burns 67–70; circular patches 153; cold and clammy 160;

hives 118–19; infected spots 120–1; infection 120–1; inflammation 149–50; itching 98–9, 156–7; measles 128–30; nappy rash 140; rash 154–5, 128–30; reddened 158–9; scaly 152; sunburn 68–70; sweating profusely 113, 160; swelling after injury 109–10; warts 184; weeping 98–9; wounds 190–3; yellow 124–7

Sleep 163–5

Sleepwalking 164–5; & anxiety 47

Slow development 48

Spasm, asthma 49–52; cramps 113–14; coughing 185–7; muscles 113–14; stomach 85–6; urination 182

Spine problems, & headaches 111

Spots and Rashes 166–7

Sprains 168–9

Squint 103

Stings 57–9; & hives 118–19

Stomach, cramps 85–6

Strains 168–9

Stress, and headache 111–12 (*see also* Anxiety)

Stye 101–2

Sucking, in babies 53–4

Sugar, in blood 111

Sunburn 68–70

Sunstroke 113

Swallowing, difficulties 177–9

Swelling, ankles 42; bruise 66; ear, under 138–9; fractures 109–10; glands 154, 159, 177–9; groin 197–9; injury, after 109–10; jaw, under 174; neck 159, 177–9; end of penis 196–7; skin, abscess 33–4, boils 61–2; sprains 168–9 ; testicle 197–8

Syrup, herbal 17

Tantrums *see* Anxiety

Tear duct, blocked 102

Teeth, ache 171–2; decay 171; grinding 188–9; teething 170

Temperature, *see* Fever

Tendon, strain 168–9

Testicle, fluid around 197–8; swollen 139, 196–8; undescended 198

Throat **173–4**; fiery red 158–9; larynx 87–8; obstruction 73; repeated infection 173–4; scratched 74; sore 63–5, 122–3, 128

Thrush **175–6**; in babies 54

Toothache, *see* Teeth

Tonsils 177–9

Travel sickness 180–1

Tummy button, *see* Navel

Ulcers, mouth 137

Umbilical cord, infection 53, 55, 124

Unconsciousness, after heatstroke 113–14

Urine, in babies 55; cystitis 182–3; discoloration 124–7; frequency 45; pain on urination 196–7; urinary tract infection 182–3

Urticaria 118–19

Vaccination 31–2; & resistance 30–1

Vagina, discharge 175–6; infection 175–6; itching 175–6, 188–9

Visual disturbances 103, 128; blurred 103; poor vision 102–3

Vomiting, in babies 54; & heatstroke 113–14; & travel 183–4; & scarlet fever 158–9; & shock 160